Intermittent Fasting Recipes

Kitchen-Tested Recipes to Quickly Shed Those Stubborn Pounds and Save Time and Money

Delilah Roman

Valor Cooking Publishing

CONTENTS

Ground Beef with Veggies

Prep time: 15 minutes | Cook time: 25 minutes | Serves 4

1 pound (454 g) lean ground beef

2 tablespoons extra-virgin olive oil

2 garlic cloves, minced

½ yellow onion, chopped

2 cups fresh mushrooms, sliced

1 cup fresh kale, tough ribs removed and chopped

¼ cup low-sodium beef broth

2 tablespoons balsamic vinegar

2 tablespoons fresh parsley, chopped

1. Heat a large nonstick skillet over medium-high heat and cook the ground beef for about 8 to 10 minutes, breaking up the chunks with a wooden spoon.
2. With a slotted spoon, transfer the beef into a bowl.
3. In the same skillet, add the onion and garlic for about 3 minutes.
4. Add the mushrooms and cook for about 5 minutes.
5. Add the cooked beef, kale, broth and vinegar and bring to a boil.
6. Reduce the heat to medium-low and simmer for about 3 minutes.
7. Stir in parsley and serve immediately.

Fish and Spinach Curry

Prep time: 15 minutes | Cook time: 15 minutes | Serves 4

1 tablespoon coconut oil

1 small yellow onion, chopped

2 garlic cloves, minced

1 teaspoon fresh ginger, minced

1 large tomato, peeled and chopped

1 tablespoon curry powder

¼ cup water

1¼ cups unsweetened coconut milk

1 pound (454 g) skinless grouper fillets, cubed into 2-inch size

¾ pound (340 g) fresh spinach, chopped

Salt, to taste

2 tablespoons fresh parsley, chopped

1. In a large wok, melt the coconut oil over medium heat and sauté the onion, garlic and ginger for about 5 minutes.
2. Add the tomatoes and curry powder and cook for about 2 to 3 minutes, crushing with the back of spoon.
3. Add the water and coconut milk and bring to a gentle boil.
4. Stir in grouper pieces and spinach and cook for about 4 to 5 minutes.
5. Stir in the salt and parsley and serve hot.

Pork and Veggie Burgers

Prep time: 15 minutes | Cook time: 16 minutes | Serves 4

Patties:

1 pound (454 g) ground pork

1 carrot, peeled and chopped finely

1 medium raw beetroot, trimmed, peeled and chopped finely

1 small onion, chopped finely

2 Serrano peppers, seeded and chopped

1 tablespoon fresh cilantro, chopped finely

Salt and ground black pepper, to taste

3 tablespoons olive oil

Burgers:

1 large onion, sliced

2 large tomatoes, sliced

4 lettuce leaves

1. For patties: In a large bowl, add all ingredients except for oil and mix until well combined.
2. Make equal-sized 8 patties from the mixture.
3. In a large nonstick sauté pan, heat the olive oil over medium heat and cook the patties in 2 batches for about 3 to 4 minutes per side or until golden brown.
4. Arrange the bun bottoms onto serving plates.
5. Plce1 patty over each bun, followed by the onion, tomato and lettuce.
6. Cover each with top of bun and serve.

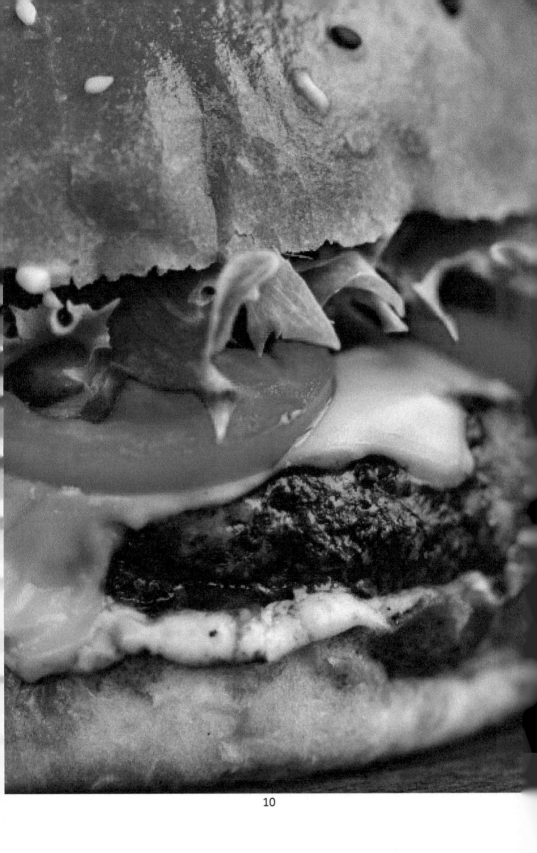

Chicken and Strawberry Lettuce Wraps

Prep time: 15 minutes | Cook time: 0 minutes | Serves 2

6 ounces (170 g) cooked chicken breast, cut into strips

½ cup fresh strawberries, hulled and sliced thinly

1 English cucumber, sliced thinly

1 tablespoon fresh mint leaves, minced

4 large lettuce leaves

1. In a large bowl, add all ingredients except lettuce leaves and gently toss to coat well.
2. Place the lettuce leaves onto serving plates.
3. Place the chicken mixture over each lettuce leaf evenly and serve immediately.

Beef Lettuce Wraps

Prep time: 15 minutes | Cook time: 13 minutes | Serves 2

2 tablespoons white onion, chopped

5 ounces (142 g) lean ground beef

2 tablespoons light thousand island dressing

⅛ teaspoon white vinegar

⅛ teaspoon onion powder

4 lettuce leaves

2 tablespoons low-fat Cheddar cheese, shredded

1 small cucumber, julienned

1. Heat a small, lightly greased skillet over medium-high heat and sauté the onion for about 2 to 3 minutes.
2. Add the beef and cook for about 8 to 10 minutes or until cooked through.
3. Remove from the heat and set aside.
4. In a bowl, add the dressing, vinegar and onion powder and mix well.
5. Arrange the lettuce leaves onto serving plates.
6. Place beef mixture over each lettuce leaf, followed by the cheese and cucumber.
7. Drizzle with sauce and serve.

Tempeh with Bell Peppers

Prep time: 15 minutes | Cook time: 15 minutes | Serves 3

2 tablespoons balsamic vinegar

2 tablespoons low-sodium soy sauce

2 tablespoons tomato sauce

1 teaspoon maple syrup

½ teaspoon garlic powder

⅛ teaspoon red pepper flakes, crushed

1 tablespoon vegetable oil

8 ounces (227 g) tempeh, cut into cubes

1 medium onion, chopped

2 large green bell peppers, seeded and chopped

1. In a small bowl, add the vinegar, soy sauce, tomato sauce, maple syrup, garlic powder and red pepper flakes and beat until well combined. Set aside.
2. Heat 1 tablespoon of oil in a large skillet over medium heat and cook the tempeh about 2 to 3 minutes per side.
3. Add the onion and bell peppers and heat for about 2 to 3 minutes.
4. Stir in the sauce mixture and cook for about 3 to 5 minutes, stirring frequently.
5. Serve hot.

Vegetarian Burgers

Prep time: 15 minutes | Cook time: 16 minutes | Serves 4

1 pound (454 g) firm tofu, drained, pressed, and crumbled

¾ cup rolled oats

¼ cup flaxseeds

2 cups frozen spinach, thawed

1 medium onion, chopped finely

4 garlic cloves, minced

1 teaspoon ground cumin

1 teaspoon red pepper flakes, crushed

Sea salt and freshly ground black pepper, to taste

2 tablespoons olive oil

6 cups fresh salad greens

1. In a large bowl, add all the ingredients except oil and salad greens and mix until well combined.
2. Set aside for about 10 minutes.
3. Make desired size patties from the mixture.
4. In a nonstick frying pan, heat the oil over medium heat and cook the patties for 6 to 8 minutes per side.
5. Serve these patties alongside the salad greens.

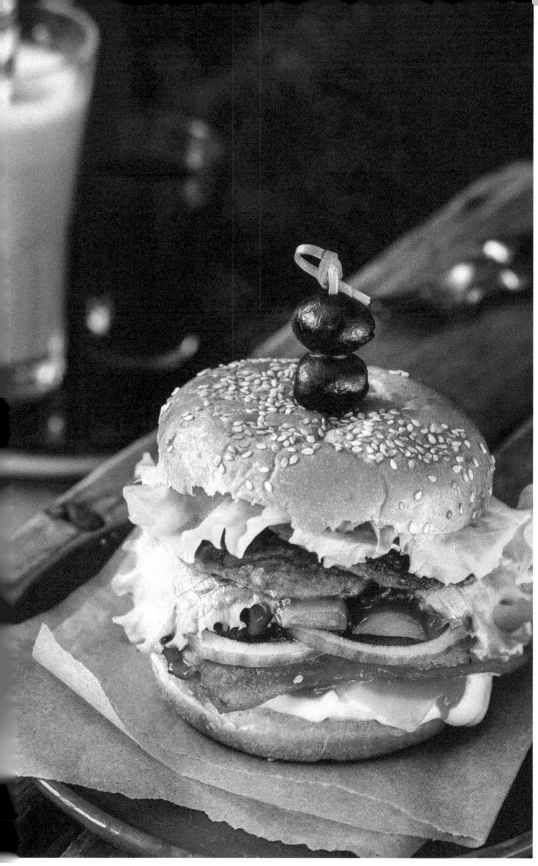

Garlicky Beef Tenderloin

Prep time: 10 minutes | Cook time: 50 minutes | Serves 19

1 (3-pound / 1.4-kg) center-cut beef tenderloin roast

4 garlic cloves, minced

1 tablespoon fresh rosemary, minced

Salt and ground black pepper, to taste

1 tablespoon olive oil

15 cups fresh spinach

1. Preheat the oven to 425°F (220°C).
2. Grease a large shallow roasting pan.
3. Place the roast into the prepared roasting pan.
4. Rub the roast with garlic, rosemary, salt, and black pepper, and drizzle with oil.
5. Roast the beef for about 45 to 50 minutes.
6. Remove from oven and place the roast onto a cutting board for about 10 minutes.
7. With a knife, cut beef tenderloin into desired-sized slices and serve alongside the spinach.

Turkey Chili

Prep time: 15 minutes | Cook time: 2¼ hours | Serves 8

2 tablespoons olive oil

1 small yellow onion, chopped

1 green bell pepper, seeded and chopped

4 garlic cloves, minced

1 jalapeño pepper, chopped

1 teaspoon dried thyme, crushed

2 tablespoons red chili powder

1 tablespoon ground cumin

2 pounds (907 g) lean ground turkey

2 cups fresh tomatoes, chopped finely

2 ounces (57 g) sugar-free tomato paste

2 cups homemade low-sodium chicken broth

1 cup water

Salt and ground black pepper, to taste

1. In a large Dutch oven, heat oil over medium heat and sauté the onion and bell pepper for about 5 to 7 minutes.
2. Add the garlic, jalapeño pepper, thyme and spices and sauté for about 1 minute.
3. Add the turkey and cook for about 4 to 5 minutes.
4. Stir in the tomatoes, tomato paste and cacao powder and cook for about 2 minutes.
5. Add in the broth and water and bring to a boil.
6. Now, reduce the heat to low and simmer, covered for about 2 hours.

7. Add in salt and black pepper and remove from the heat.

8. Serve hot.

Bok Choy and Mushroom Stir-Fry

Prep time: 15 minutes | Cook time: 10 minutes | Serves 4

1 pound (454 g) baby bok choy

4 teaspoons olive oil

1 teaspoon fresh ginger, minced

2 garlic cloves, chopped

5 ounces (142 g) fresh mushrooms, sliced

2 tablespoons red wine

2 tablespoons soy sauce

Ground black pepper, to taste

1. Trim bases of bok choy and separate outer leaves from stalks, leaving the smallest inner leaves attached.

2. In a large cast-iron wok, heat the oil over medium-high heat and sauté the ginger and garlic for about 1 minute.

3. Stir in the mushrooms and cook for about 4 to 5 minutes, stirring frequently.

4. Stir in the bok choy leaves and stalks and cook for about 1 minute, tossing with tongs.

5. Stir in the wine, soy sauce and black pepper and cook for about 2 to 3 minutes, tossing occasionally.

6. Serve hot.

Roasted Mackerel

Prep time: 10 minutes | Cook time: 20 minutes | Serves 2

2 (7-ounce / 198-g) mackerel fillets

1 tablespoon olive oil

Salt and ground black pepper, to taste

3 cups fresh baby greens

1. Preheat the oven to 350°F (180°C).
2. Arrange a rack in the middle of oven.
3. Lightly grease a baking dish.
4. Brush the fish fillets with melted butter and then season with salt and black pepper.
5. Arrange the fish fillets into the prepared baking dish in a single layer.
6. Bake for approximately 20 minutes.
7. Serve hot alongside the greens.

Squash Casserole

Prep time: 15 minutes | Cook time: 55 minutes | Serves 8

¼ cup plus 2 tablespoons olive oil, divided

1 small yellow onion, chopped

3 summer squashes, sliced

4 eggs, beaten

3 cups low-fat Cheddar cheese, shredded and divided

2 tablespoons unsweetened almond milk

2 to 3 tablespoons almond flour

2 tablespoons erythritol

Salt and ground black pepper, to taste

1. Preheat the oven to 375°F (190°C).
2. In a large skillet, heat 2 tablespoons of oil over medium heat and cook the onion and squash for about 8 to 10 minutes, stirring occasionally.
3. Remove the skillet from the heat.
4. Place the eggs, 1 cup of Cheddar cheese, almond milk, almond flour, erythritol, salt and black pepper in a large bowl and mix until well combined.
5. Add the squash mixture, and remaining oil and stir to combine.
6. Transfer the mixture into a large casserole dish and sprinkle with the remaining Cheddar cheese.
7. Bake for approximately 35 to 45 minutes.
8. Remove the casserole dish from oven and set aside for about 5 to 10 minutes before serving.
9. Cut into 8 equal-sized portions and serve.

Beef and Broccoli Bowl

Prep time: 15 minutes | Cook time: 12 minutes | Serves 1

4 ounces (113 g) lean ground beef

1 cup broccoli, cut into bite-sized pieces

2 tablespoons low-sodium chicken broth

¼ cup tomatoes, chopped

¼ teaspoon onion powder

¼ teaspoon garlic powder

Pinch of red pepper flakes

Salt, to taste

1 ounce (28 g) low-fat Cheddar cheese

1. Heat a lightly greased skillet over medium heat and cook the beef for about 8 to 10 minutes or until browned completely.
2. Meanwhile, in a microwave-safe bowl, place the broccoli and broth.
3. With a plastic wrap, cover the bowl and microwave for about 4 minutes.
4. Remove from the microwave and set aside.
5. Drain the grease from skillet.
6. Add the tomatoes, garlic powder, onion powder, red pepper flakes and salt and stir to combine well.
7. Add the broccoli and toss to coat well.
8. Remove from the heat and transfer the beef mixture into a serving bowl.
9. Top with Cheddar cheese and serve.

Tofu and Veggie Lettuce Wraps

Prep time: 15 minutes | Cook time: 6 minutes | Serves 4

Wraps:

1 tablespoon olive oil

14 ounces (397 g) extra-firm tofu, drained, pressed and cut into cubes

1 teaspoon curry powder

Salt, to taste

8 lettuce leaves

1 small carrot, peeled and julienned

½ cup radishes, sliced

2 tablespoons fresh cilantro, chopped

Sauce:

½ cup creamy peanut butter

1 tablespoon maple syrup

2 tablespoons low-sodium soy sauce

2 tablespoons fresh lime juice

¼ teaspoon red pepper flakes, crushed

¼ cup water

1. For tofu: In a skillet, heat the oil over medium heat and cook the tofu, curry powder and a little salt for about 5 to 6 minutes or until golden brown, stirring frequently.
2. Remove from the heat and set aside to cool slightly.
3. Meanwhile, for sauce: In a bowl, add all the ingredients and beat until smooth.
4. Arrange the lettuce leaves onto serving plates.
5. Divide the tofu, carrot, radish and peanuts over each leaf evenly.
6. Garnish with cilantro and serve alongside the peanut sauce.

Mini Bacon Cheeseburger Bites

Prep time: 10 minutes | Cook time: 18 minutes | Serves 4

1 pound (454 g) lean ground beef

¼ cup finely chopped yellow onion

1 tablespoon Worcestershire sauce

1 tablespoon yellow mustard

1 clove garlic, minced

½ teaspoon salt

Cooking spray

4 ultra-thin slices Cheddar cheese, each cut into 6 equal-sized rectangular pieces

3 pieces cooked turkey bacon, each cut into 8 equal-sized rectangular pieces

24 dill pickle chips

4 to 6 large green leaf lettuce leaves, torn into 24 (total) small square-shaped pieces

12 cherry tomatoes, sliced in half

1. Preheat the oven to 400°F (205°C). Line a baking sheet with aluminum foil.
2. In a medium mixing bowl, stir together the ground beef, onion, Worcestershire sauce, mustard, garlic, and salt until well mixed. Shape the mixture into 24 small meatballs. Arrange the meatballs on the prepared baking sheet and spray them with cooking spray.
3. Bake in the preheated oven for about 15 minutes until cooked through.

4. Place a piece of cheese on top of each meatball and bake for an additional 2 to 3 minutes, or until the cheese is melted. Remove from the oven and let cool.

5. Assemble the bites: On a toothpick, layer a cheese-covered meatball, piece of bacon, pickle chip, piece of lettuce, and cherry tomato half, in that order. Serve immediately.

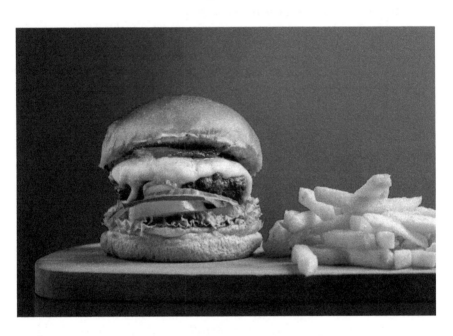

Tofu with Peas

Prep time: 15 minutes | Cook time: 20 minutes | Serves 5

2 tablespoons olive oil, divided

1 (16-ounce / 454-g) package extra-firm tofu, drained, pressed and cubed

1 cup yellow onion, chopped

1 tablespoon fresh ginger, minced

2 garlic cloves, minced

1 tomato, chopped finely

2 cups frozen peas, thawed

¼ cup water

2 tablespoons fresh cilantro, chopped

1. In a nonstick wok, heat 1 tablespoon of the oil over medium-high heat and cook the tofu for about 4 to 5 minutes or until browned completely, stirring occasionally.
2. Transfer the tofu into a bowl.
3. In the same wok, heat the remaining oil over medium heat and sauté the onion for about 3 to 4 minutes.
4. Add the ginger and garlic and sauté for about 1 minute.
5. Add the tomatoes and cook for about 4 to 5 minutes, crushing with the back of a spoon.
6. Stir in the peas and broth and cook for about 2 to 3 minutes.
7. Stir in the tofu and cook for about 1 to 2 minutes.
8. Serve hot with the garnishing of cilantro.

Cheesy Mushroom Soup

Prep time: 15 minutes | Cook time: 15 minutes | Serves 4

2 tablespoons olive oil

4 ounces (113 g) fresh baby portobello mushroom, sliced

4 ounces (113 g) fresh white button mushrooms, sliced

½ cup yellow onion, chopped

½ teaspoon salt

1 teaspoon garlic, chopped

3 cups low-sodium vegetable broth

1 cup low-fat Cheddar cheese

1. In a medium pan, heat the oil over medium heat and cook the mushrooms and onion with salt for about 5 to 7 minutes, stirring frequently.
2. Add the garlic, and sauté for about 1 to 2 minutes.
3. Stir in the broth and remove from the heat.
4. With a stick blender, blend the soup until mushrooms are chopped very finely.
5. In the pan, add the heavy cream and stir to combine.
6. Place the pan over medium heat and cook for about 3 to 5 minutes.
7. Remove from the heat and serve immediately.

Prawns with Asparagus

Prep time: 15 minutes | Cook time: 13 minutes | Serves 4

3 tablespoons extra-virgin olive oil

1 pound (454 g) prawns, peeled and deveined

1 pound (454 g) asparagus, trimmed

Salt and ground black pepper, to taste

1 teaspoon garlic, minced

1 teaspoon fresh ginger, minced

1 tablespoon low-sodium soy sauce

2 tablespoons lemon juice

1. In a wok, heat 2 tablespoons of oil over medium-high heat and cook the prawns with salt and black pepper for about 3 to 4 minutes.
2. With a slotted spoon, transfer the prawns into a bowl. Set aside.
3. In the same wok, heat remaining 1 tablespoon of oil over medium-high heat and cook the asparagus, ginger, garlic, salt and black pepper and for about 6 to 8 minutes, stirring frequently.
4. Stir in the prawns and soy sauce and cook for about 1 minute.
5. Stir in the lemon juice and remove from the heat.
6. Serve hot.

Balsamic Chicken Breast

Prep time: 10 minutes | Cook time: 14 minutes | Serves 4

¼ cup balsamic vinegar

2 tablespoons olive oil

1½ teaspoons fresh lemon juice

½ teaspoon lemon-pepper seasoning

4 (6-ounce / 170-g) boneless, skinless chicken breast halves, pounded slightly

6 cups fresh baby kale

1. In a glass baking dish, place the vinegar, oil, lemon juice and seasoning and mix well.
2. Add the chicken breasts and coat with the mixture generously.
3. Refrigerate to marinate for about 25 to 30 minutes.
4. Preheat the grill to medium heat.
5. Grease the grill grate.
6. Remove the chicken from bowl and discard the remaining marinade.
7. Place the chicken breasts onto the grill and cover with the lid.
8. Cook for about 5 to 7 minutes per side or until desired doneness.
9. Serve hot alongside the kale.

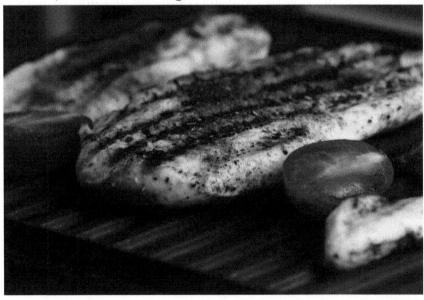

Shrimp and Scallops with Veggies

Prep time: 20 minutes | Cook time: 11 minutes | Serves 5

3 tablespoons olive oil, divided

1 pound (454 g) fresh asparagus, cut into 2-inch pieces

2 red bell peppers, seeded and chopped

¾ pound (340 g) medium raw shrimp, peeled and deveined

¾ pound (340 g) raw scallops

1 tablespoon dried parsley

½ teaspoon garlic, minced

Salt and freshly ground black pepper, to taste

1. In a large skillet, heat 1 tablespoon of oil over medium heat and stir-fry the asparagus and bell peppers for about 4 to 5 minutes.
2. With a slotted spoon, transfer the vegetables onto a plate.
3. In the same skillet, heat the remaining oil over medium heat and stir-fry shrimp and scallops for about 2 minutes.
4. Stir in the parsley, garlic, salt, and black pepper, and cook for about 1 minute.
5. Add in the cooked vegetables and cook for about 2 to 3 minutes.
6. Serve hot.

Tofu and Mushroom Soup

Prep time: 15 minutes | Cook time: 25 minutes | Serves 3

3 tablespoons vegetable oil, divided

1 shallot, minced

1 ounce (28 g) fresh ginger, minced

2 garlic cloves, minced

5½ ounces (156 g) coconut milk

1 Roma tomato, chopped

1 lemongrass stalk, halved crosswise

6 ounces (170 g) fresh mushrooms, sliced

14 ounces (397 g) extra-firm tofu, pressed, drained and cut into ½-inch cubes

Ground black pepper, to taste

1 scallion, sliced

1 tablespoon fresh cilantro

1. In a pan, heat 2 tablespoons of oil over medium-high heat and sauté the shallot, ginger, garlic and a pinch of salt for about 1 to 2 minutes.
2. Add coconut milk and remaining water and bring to a boil.
3. Add the tomato and lemongrass and stir to combine.
4. Adjust the heat to low and simmer for about 8 to 10 minutes.
5. Meanwhile, in a large nonstick skillet, heat the remaining oil over medium-high heat and cook the mushrooms, tofu, pinch of salt and black pepper for about 5 to 8 minutes, stirring occasionally.

6. Remove the lemongrass stalk from pan of soup and discard it.

7. Divide the cooked mushrooms and tofu into serving bowls evenly.

8. Top with hot soup and serve with the garnishing of cilantro.

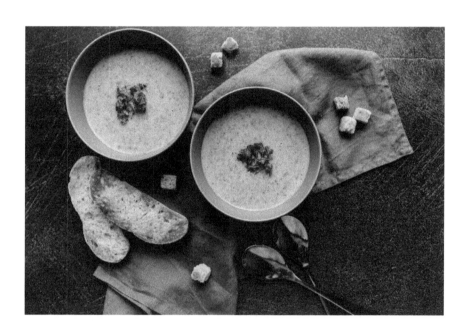

Scallops with Spinach

Prep time: 15 minutes | Cook time: 21 minutes | Serves 5

1 tablespoon olive oil

1½ pounds (680 g) jumbo sea scallops

Salt and ground black pepper, to taste

1 cup onion, chopped

6 garlic cloves, minced

14 ounces (397 g) fresh baby spinach

1. In a large nonstick skillet, heat the oil over medium-high heat and cook the scallops with salt and black pepper for about 5 minutes, turning once after 2½ minutes.
2. Transfer the scallops into another bowl and cover them with a piece of foil to keep warm.
3. In the same skillet, add onion and garlic over medium heat and sauté the onion and garlic for about 3 minutes.
4. Add the spinach and cook for about 2 to 3 minutes.
5. Season with salt and black pepper and remove from the heat.
6. Divide the spinach onto serving plates.
7. Top with scallops and serve immediately.

Tuna Stuffed Avocado

Prep time: 15 minutes | Cook time: 0 minutes | Serves 2

1 large avocado, halved and pitted

1 tablespoon onion, chopped finely

2 tablespoons fresh lemon juice

5 ounces (142 g) cooked tuna, chopped

Salt and ground black pepper, to taste

1. With a spoon, scoop out the flesh from the middle of each avocado half and transfer into a bowl.
2. Add the onion and lemon juice and mash until well combined.
3. Add tuna, salt and black pepper and stir to combine.
4. Divide the tuna mixture in both avocado halves evenly and serve immediately.

Turkey Stuffed Acorn Squash

Prep time: 15 minutes | Cook time: 50 minutes | Serves 4

2 acorn squash, halved and seeded

1 pound (454 g) lean ground turkey breast

1 cup red onion, chopped

1 cup celery stalk, chopped

1 cup fresh button mushrooms, sliced

8 ounces (227 g) sugar-free tomato sauce

1 teaspoon dried oregano, crushed

1 teaspoon dried basil, crushed

Freshly ground black pepper, to taste

1 cup low-fat Cheddar cheese, shredded

1. Preheat the oven to 350°F (180°C).
2. In the bottom of a microwave-safe glass baking dish, arrange the squash halves, cut side down.
3. Microwave on High for about 20 minutes or until almost tender.
4. Heat a large nonstick skillet over medium heat and cook the ground turkey for about 4 to 5 minutes or until meat is no longer pink.
5. Drain the grease completely.
6. Add the onion and celery and cook for about 3 to 4 minutes.
7. Stir in the mushrooms and cook for about 2 to 3 minutes more.
8. Stir in the tomato sauce, dried herbs and black pepper and remove from the heat.
9. Spoon the turkey mixture into each squash half.
10. Cover the baking dish and bake for about 15 minutes.
11. Uncover the baking dish and sprinkle each squash half with Cheddar cheese.
12. Bake uncovered for about 3 to 5 minutes or until the cheese becomes bubbly.
13. Serve hot.

Shrimp Kabobs

Prep time: 15 minutes | Cook time: 8 minutes | Serves 3

¼ cup olive oil

2 tablespoons fresh lime juice

½ chipotle pepper in adobo sauce, seeded and minced

1 garlic cloves, minced

1½ teaspoon powdered erythritol

½ teaspoon red chili powder

½ teaspoon paprika

¼ teaspoon ground cumin

Salt and ground black pepper, to taste

1 pound (454 g) medium raw shrimp, peeled and deveined

5 cups fresh salad greens

1. In a bowl, add all the ingredients except the shrimp and greens and mix well.
2. Add the shrimp and coat with the herb mixture generously.
3. Refrigerate to marinate for at least 30 minutes.
4. Preheat the grill to medium-high heat.
5. Grease the grill grate.
6. Thread the shrimp onto the re soaked wooden skewers.
7. Place the skewers onto the grill and cook for about 3 to 4 minutes per side.
8. Remove from the grill and place onto a platter for about 5 minutes before serving.

Prawns with Broccoli

Prep time: 20 minutes | Cook time: 10 minutes | Serves 4

2 tablespoons olive oil, divided

1 pound (454 g) large prawns, peeled and deveined

½ onion, chopped

3 garlic cloves, minced

3 cups broccoli floret

2 tablespoons low-sodium soy sauce

Freshly ground black pepper, to taste

2 tablespoons fresh parsley, chopped

1. In a large nonstick skillet, heat 1 tablespoon of olive oil over medium heat and stir-fry the prawns for about 1 minute per side.
2. With a slotted spoon, transfer the prawns onto a plate.
3. In the same skillet, heat the remaining oil over medium heat and sauté the onion and garlic for about 2 to 3 minutes.
4. Add the broccoli, soy sauce and black pepper and stir-fry for about 2 to 3 minutes.
5. Stir in the cooked prawns and stir-fry for about 1 to 2 minutes.
6. Serve hot.

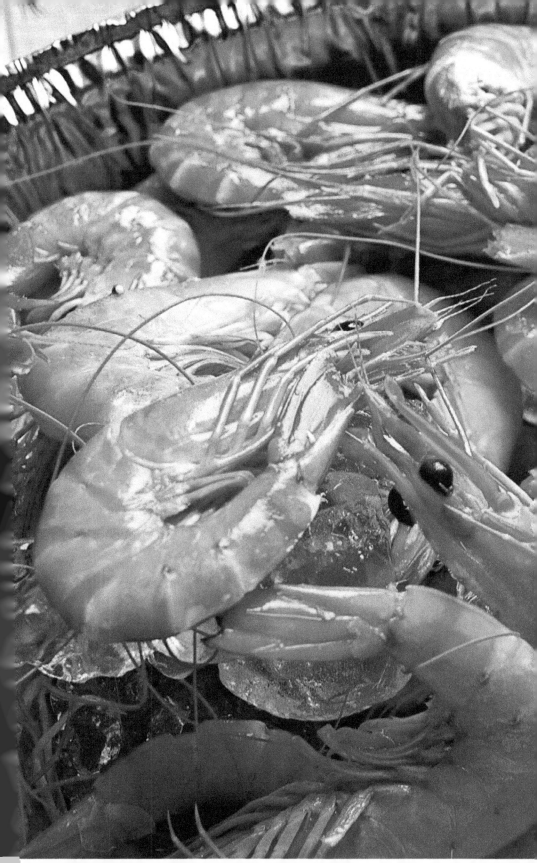

Blueberries and Spinach Salad

Prep time: 15 minutes | Cook time: 0 minutes | Serves 4

Salad:

6 cups fresh baby spinach

1½ cups fresh blueberries

¼ cup onion, sliced

¼ cup almond, sliced

¼ cup feta cheese, crumbled

Dressing:

⅓ cup olive oil

2 tablespoons fresh lemon juice

¼ teaspoon liquid stevia

⅛ teaspoon garlic powder

Salt, to taste

1. For salad: In a bowl, add the spinach, berries, onion and almonds and mix.
2. For dressing: In another small bowl, add all the ingredients and beat until well blended.
3. Place the dressing over salad and gently toss to coat well.
4. Serve immediately.

Orange Chicken

Prep time: 10 minutes | Cook time: 20 minutes | Serves 6

3 garlic cloves, minced

½ cup fresh orange juice

1 tablespoon apple cider vinegar

2 tablespoons low-sodium soy sauce

¼ teaspoon ground ginger

¼ teaspoon ground cinnamon

Freshly ground black pepper, to taste

2 pounds (907 g) skinless, bone-in chicken thighs

⅓ cup scallion, sliced

1. For marinade: In a large bowl, mix together all ingredients except for chicken thighs and scallion.
2. Add the chicken thighs and coat with marinade generously.
3. Cover the bowl and refrigerate to marinate for about 4 hours.
4. Remove the chicken from bowl, reserving marinade.
5. Heat a lightly greased large nonstick skillet over medium-high heat and cook the chicken thighs for about 5 to 6 minutes or till golden brown.
6. Flip the side and cook for about 4 minutes.
7. Stir in the reserved marinade and bring to a boil.
8. Reduce the heat to medium-low and cook, covered for about 6 to 8 minutes or until sauce becomes thick.
9. Stir in the scallion and remove from the heat.

10. Serve hot.

Zesty Salmon

Prep time: 10 minutes | Cook time: 10 minutes | Serves 4

1 tablespoon butter, melted

1 tablespoon fresh lemon juice

1 teaspoon Worcestershire sauce

1 teaspoon lemon zest, grated finely.

4 (6-ounce / 170-g) salmon fillets

Salt and ground black pepper, to taste

1. In a baking dish, place butter, lemon juice, Worcestershire sauce, and lemon zest, and mix well.
2. Coat the fillets with mixture and then arrange skin side-up in the baking dish.
3. Set aside for about 15 minutes.
4. Preheat the broiler of oven.
5. Arrange the oven rack about 6-inch from heating element.
6. Line a broiler pan with a piece of foil.
7. Remove the salmon fillets from baking dish and season with salt and black pepper.
8. Arrange the salmon fillets onto the prepared broiler pan, skin side down.
9. Broil for about 8 to 10 minutes.
10. Serve hot.

Chicken and Cauliflower Curry

Prep time: 15 minutes | Cook time: 20 minutes | Serves 6

¼ cup olive oil

3 garlic cloves, minced

2 tablespoons curry powder

1½ pounds (680 g) skinless, boneless chicken thighs, cut into bite-sized pieces

Salt and ground black pepper, to taste

1 pound (454 g) cauliflower, cut into small pieces

1 green bell pepper, seeded and chopped

14 ounces (397 g) unsweetened coconut milk

¼ cup fresh parsley, chopped

1. In a large skillet, heat the oil over medium heat and sauté the garlic and curry powder for about 1 minute.
2. Add the chicken, salt and black pepper and cook for about 5 to 6 minutes, stirring frequently.
3. With a slotted spoon, transfer the chicken onto a plate.
4. In the skillet, add the cauliflower and bell pepper and cook for about 2 to 3 minutes.
5. Add the coconut milk and simmer for about 5 to 7 minutes.
6. Stir in the cooked chicken, salt and black pepper and cook for about 2 to 3 minutes.
7. Serve hot with the garnishing of parsley.

Lemony Chicken Thighs

Prep time: 10 minutes | Cook time: 16 minutes | Serves 4

2 tablespoons olive oil, divided

1 tablespoon fresh lemon juice

1 tablespoon lemon zest, grated

2 teaspoons dried oregano

1 teaspoon dried thyme

Salt and ground black pepper, to taste

1½ pounds (680 g) bone-in chicken thighs

6 cups fresh baby spinach

1. Preheat the oven to 425°F (220°C).
2. Add 1 tablespoon of the oil, lemon juice, lemon zest, dried herbs, salt, and black pepper in a large mixing bowl and mix well.
3. Add the chicken thighs and coat with the mixture generously.
4. Refrigerate to marinate for at least 20 minutes.
5. In an oven-proof wok, heat the remaining oil over medium-high heat and sear the chicken thighs for about 2 to 3 minutes per side.
6. Immediately transfer the wok into the oven and Bake for approximately 10 minutes.
7. Serve hot alongside the spinach.

Steak with Green Beans

Prep time: 15 minutes | Cook time: 10 minutes | Serves 2

Steak:

2 (5-ounce / 142-g) sirloin steaks, trimmed

Salt and ground black pepper, to taste

1 tablespoon extra-virgin olive oil

1 garlic clove, minced

Green Beans:

½ pound (227 g) fresh green beans

½ tablespoon olive oil

½ tablespoon fresh lemon juice

1. For steak: Season the steaks with salt and black pepper evenly.
2. In a cast iron sauté pan, heat the olive oil over high heat and sauté garlic for about 15 to 20 seconds.
3. Add the steaks and cook for about 3 minutes per side.
4. Flip the steaks and cook for about 3 to 4 minutes or until desired doneness, flipping once.
5. Meanwhile, for green beans: In a pan of boiling water, arrange a steamer basket.
6. Place the green beans in a steamer basket and steam covered for about 4 to 5 minutes.
7. Carefully transfer the beans into a bowl.
8. Add olive oil and lemon juice and toss to coat well.
9. Divide green beans onto serving plates.
10. Top each with 1 steak and serve.

Turkey, Apple and Veggies Burgers

Prep time: 20 minutes | Cook time: 12 minutes | Serves 4

Burgers:

12 ounces (340 g) lean ground turkey

½ apple, peeled, cored and grated

½ red bell pepper, seeded and chopped finely

¼ cup red onion, minced

2 small garlic cloves, minced

1 tablespoon fresh ginger, minced

2½ tablespoons fresh cilantro, chopped

2 tablespoons curry paste

1 teaspoon ground cumin

1 teaspoon olive oil

For Serving:

6 cups fresh baby spinach

1. Preheat the grill to medium heat. Grease the grill grate.
2. For burgers: In a large bowl, add all the ingredients except for oil and mix until well combined.
3. Make 4 equal-sized burgers from the mixture.
4. Brush the burgers with olive oil evenly.
5. Place the burgers onto the grill and cook for about 5 to 6 minutes per side.
6. Divide the baby spinach onto serving plates and top each with 1 burger.
7. Serve immediately.

Chicken and Avocado Burgers

Prep time: 15 minutes | Cook time: 10 minutes | Serves 4

½ ripe avocado, peeled, pitted and cut into chunks

½ cup low-fat Parmesan cheese, grated

1 garlic clove, minced

Freshly ground black pepper, to taste

1 pound (454 g) lean ground chicken

Olive oil cooking spray

6 cups fresh baby green

1. In a bowl, add the avocado chunks, Parmesan cheese, garlic and black pepper and toss to coat well.
2. Add the ground chicken and gently, stir to combine.
3. Make 4 equal-sized patties from the chicken mixture.
4. Heat a greased grill pan over medium heat.
5. Place the patties into grill pan and cook for about 5 minutes per side.
6. Divide the greens onto serving plates and top each with 1 burger.
7. Serve immediately.

Turkey Meatballs Kabobs

Prep time: 15 minutes | Cook time: 14 minutes | Serves 4

1 yellow onion, chopped roughly

½ cup lemongrass, chopped roughly

2 garlic cloves, chopped roughly

1½ pounds (680 g) lean ground turkey

1 teaspoon sesame oil

½ tablespoons low-sodium soy sauce

1 tablespoon arrowroot starch

⅛ teaspoons powdered stevia

Salt and ground black pepper, to taste

6 cups fresh baby spinach

1. Preheat the grill to medium-high heat.
2. Grease the grill grate.
3. In a food processor, add the onion, lemongrass and garlic and pulse until chopped finely.
4. Transfer the onion mixture into a large bowl.
5. Add the remaining ingredients except for spinach and mix until well combined.
6. Make 12 equal-sized balls from meat mixture.
7. Thread the balls onto the presoaked wooden skewers.
8. Place the skewers onto the grill and cook for about 6 to 7 minutes per side.
9. Serve hot alongside the spinach.

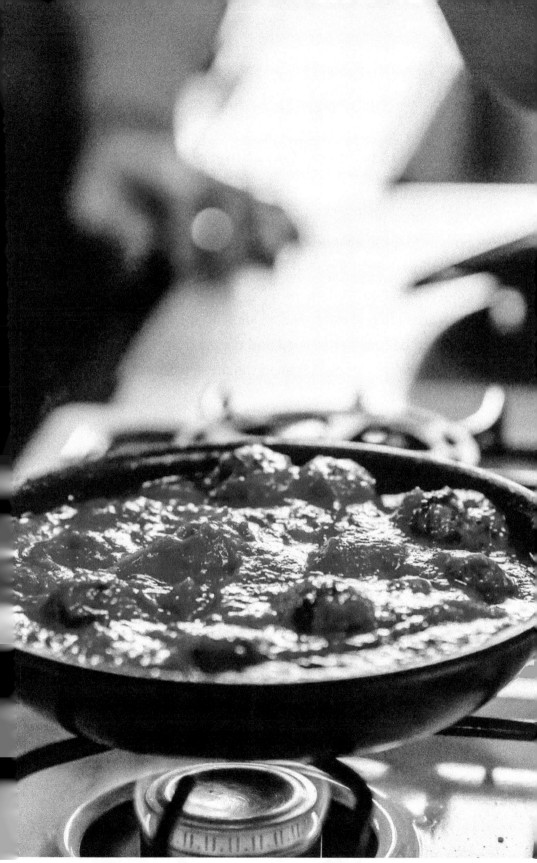

Beef Chili

Prep time: 15 minutes | Cook time: 1¾ hours | Serves 8

2 tablespoons olive oil

3 pounds (1.4 kg) ground beef

1 cup yellow onion, chopped finely

½ cup celery, chopped finely

½ cup green bell pepper, seeded and chopped finely

½ cup red bell pepper, seeded and chopped finely

1 (15-ounce / 425-g) can crushed tomatoes with juice

1½ cups tomato juice

1½ teaspoons Worcestershire sauce

½ teaspoon dried oregano

3 tablespoons red chili powder

1 teaspoon ground cumin

1 teaspoon garlic powder

1 teaspoon salt

½ teaspoon ground black pepper

1. In a large pan, heat the oil over medium-high heat and cook the beef for about 8 to 10 minutes or until browned.
2. Drain the grease from pan, leaving about 2 tablespoons inside.
3. In the pan, add the onions, celery and bell peppers over medium-high heat and cook for about 5 minutes, stirring frequently.

4. Add the tomatoes, tomato juice, Worcestershire sauce, oregano and spices and stir to combine.
5. Reduce the heat to low and simmer, covered for about 1 to 1½ hours, stirring occasionally.
6. Serve hot.

Cauliflower with Peas

Prep time: 15 minutes | Cook time: 15 minutes | Serves 4

2 medium tomatoes, chopped

¼ cup water

2 tablespoons olive oi

3 garlic cloves, minced

½ tablespoon fresh ginger, minced

1 teaspoon ground cumin

2 teaspoons ground coriander

1 teaspoon cayenne pepper

¼ teaspoon ground turmeric

2 cups cauliflower, chopped

1 cup fresh green peas, shelled

Salt and ground black pepper, to taste

½ cup warm water

1. In a blender, add tomato and ¼ cup of water and pulse until a smooth purée forms. Set aside.
2. In a large wok, heat oil over medium heat and sauté the garlic, ginger, green chilies and spices for about 1 minute.
3. Add the cauliflower, peas and tomato purée and cook, stirring for about 3 to 4 minutes.

4. Add the warm water and bring to a boil.

5. Adjust the heat to medium-low and cook, covered for about 8 to 10 minutes or until vegetables are done completely.

6. Serve hot.

Herbed Sea Bass

Prep time: 10 minutes | Cook time: 20 minutes | Serves 2

2 (1¼-pound / 567-g) whole sea bass, gutted, gilled, scaled and fins removed

Salt and ground black pepper, to taste

6 fresh bay leaves

2 fresh thyme sprigs

2 fresh parsley sprigs

2 fresh rosemary sprigs

2 tablespoons butter, melted

2 tablespoons fresh lemon juice

3 cups fresh arugula

1. Season the cavity and outer side of each fish with salt and black pepper evenly.

2. With a plastic wrap, cover each fish and refrigerate for 1 hour.

3. Preheat the oven to 450°F (235°C).

4. Lightly grease a baking dish.

5. Arrange 2 bay leaves in the bottom of the prepared baking dish.

6. Divide herb sprigs and remaining bay leaves inside the cavity of each fish.

7. Arrange both fish over bay leave in baking dish and drizzle with butter.

8. Roast for about 15 to 20 minutes or until fish is cooked through.

9. Remove the baking dish from oven and place the fish onto a platter.

10. Drizzle the fish with lemon juice and serve alongside the arugula.

Tofu with Brussels Sprout

Prep time: 15 minutes | Cook time: 15 minutes | Serves 3

1½ tablespoons olive oil, divided

8 ounces (227 g) extra-firm tofu, drained, pressed and cut into slices

2 garlic cloves, chopped

⅓ cup pecans, toasted and chopped

1 tablespoon unsweetened applesauce

¼ cup fresh cilantro, chopped

½ pound (227 g) Brussels sprouts, trimmed and cut into wide ribbons

¾ pound (340 g) mixed bell peppers, seeded and sliced

1. In a skillet, heat ½ tablespoon of the oil over medium heat and sauté the tofu and for about 6 to 7 minutes or until golden brown.

2. Add the garlic and pecans and sauté for about 1 minute.

3. Add the applesauce and cook for about 2 minutes.

4. Stir in the cilantro and remove from heat.

5. Transfer tofu into a plate and set aside

6. In the same skillet, heat the remaining oil over medium-high heat and cook the Brussels sprouts and bell peppers for about 5 minutes.

7. Stir in the tofu and remove from the heat.

8. Serve immediately.

Chicken with Yellow Squash

Prep time: 15 minutes | Cook time: 17 minutes | Serves 6

2 tablespoons olive oil, divided

1½ pounds (680 g) skinless, boneless chicken breasts, cut into bite-sized pieces

Salt and freshly ground black pepper, to taste

2 garlic cloves, minced

1½ pounds (680 g) yellow squash, sliced

2 tablespoons fresh lemon juice

1 teaspoon fresh lemon zest, grated finely

2 tablespoons fresh parsley, minced

1. In a large skillet, heat 1 tablespoon of oil over medium heat and stir-fry chicken for about 6 to 8 minutes or until golden brown from all sides.

2. Transfer the chicken onto a plate.

3. In the same skillet, heat remaining oil over medium heat and sauté garlic for about 1 minute.

4. Add the squash slices and cook for about 5 to 6 minutes,

5. Stir in the chicken and cook for about 2 minutes.

6. Stir in the lemon juice, zest and parsley and remove from heat.

7. Serve hot.

Garlicky Tilapia

Prep time: 10 minutes | Cook time: 5 minutes | Serves 4

2 tablespoons olive oil

4 (5-ounce / 142-g) tilapia fillets

3 garlic cloves, minced

1 tablespoon fresh ginger, minced

2 to 3 tablespoons low-sodium chicken broth

Salt and ground black pepper, to taste

6 cups fresh baby spinach

1. In a large sauté pan, heat the oil over medium heat and cook the tilapia fillets for about 3 minutes.
2. Flip the side and stir in the garlic and ginger.
3. Cook for about 1 to 2 minutes.
4. Add the broth and cook for about 2 to 3 more minutes.
5. Stir in salt and black pepper and remove from heat.
6. Serve hot alongside the spinach.

Bibimbap Bowls

Prep time: 10 minutes | Cook time: 12 minutes | Serves 4

1 teaspoon olive oil

5 cups baby spinach

1 teaspoon toasted sesame oil

¼ teaspoon salt

1 pound (454 g) 95 to 97% lean ground beef

1 tablespoon reduced-sodium soy sauce

2 tablespoons chili garlic sauce

2 cups riced cauliflower

1 cup thinly sliced cucumber

4 hard-boiled eggs

½ cup chopped green onions

1 tablespoon sesame seeds

1. Heat the olive oil in a skillet over medium high heat until it shimmers. Add the baby spinach and sauté for 2 to 3 minutes until just wilted. Drizzle with the sesame oil and season with salt.

2. Remove the spinach from the skillet and set aside.

3. Place the ground beef in the same skillet and cook until fully browned. Stir in the chili garlic sauce and soy sauce and cook for 1 minute. Remove the skillet from the heat and set aside.

4. Place the riced cauliflower with 1 tablespoon water in a large microwave-safe dish. Microwave on High for 3 to 4 minutes or until tender.

5. Divide ½ cup of riced cauliflower into each bowl. Top each bowl evenly with the spinach, beef, and sliced cucumber. Place an egg on top of each bowl. Serve garnished with the green onions and green onions.

Cod and Veggies Bake

Prep time: 15 minutes | Cook time: 20 minutes | Serves 4

1 teaspoon olive oil

½ cup onion, minced

1 cup zucchini, chopped

1 garlic clove, minced

2 tablespoons fresh basil, chopped

2 cups fresh tomatoes, chopped

Salt and ground black pepper, to taste

4 (6-ounce / 170-g) cod steaks

⅓ cup feta cheese, crumbled

1. Preheat the oven to 450°F (235°C).
2. Grease a large shallow baking dish.
3. In a skillet, heat oil over medium heat and sauté the onion, zucchini and garlic for about 4 to 5 minutes.
4. Stir in the basil, tomatoes, salt and black pepper and immediately remove from heat.
5. Place the cod steaks into prepared baking dish in a single layer and top with tomato mixture evenly.
6. Sprinkle with the cheese evenly.
7. Bake for approximately 15 minutes or until desired doneness.
8. Serve hot.

Steak with Carrot and Kale

Prep time: 15 minutes | Cook time: 12 minutes | Serves 4

2 tablespoons olive oil

4 garlic cloves, minced

1 pound (454 g) beef sirloin steak, cut into bite-sized pieces

Freshly ground black pepper, to taste

1½ cups carrots, peeled and cut into matchsticks

1½ cups fresh kale, tough ribs removed and chopped

3 tablespoons low-sodium soy sauce

1. In a skillet, heat the oil over medium heat and sauté the garlic for about 1 minute.
2. Add the beef and black pepper and stir to combine.
3. Increase the heat to medium-high and cook for about 3 to 4 minutes or until browned from all sides.
4. Add the carrot, kale and soy sauce and cook for about 4 to 5 minutes.
5. Stir in the black pepper and remove from the heat.
6. Serve hot.

Prep time: 10 minutes | Cook time: 20 to 25 minutes | Serves 4

4 sachets Indonesian Cinnamon and Honey Hot Cereal

½ teaspoon baking powder

1 cup unsweetened almond milk

3 tablespoons egg whites

1½ ounces (43 g) chopped pecans

¼ teaspoon cinnamon

Cooking spray

Special Equipment:

4 (4.2-ounce / 125-ml) mini mason jars

1. Preheat the oven to 350°F (180°C).
2. Combine the Indonesian Cinnamon and Honey Hot Cereal and baking powder in a bowl. Stir in the almond milk and egg white. Fold in the pecans.
3. Spritz 4 mason jars with cooking spray. Divide the mixture evenly between the jars, leaving 2 inches at the top. Sprinkle with cinnamon.
4. Bake in the preheated oven for 20 to 25 minutes on a baking sheet or until golden.
5. Allow to cool. Close the lid, refrigerate, and serve chilled.

Snack Mix

Prep time: 5 minutes | Cook time: 0 minutes | Serves 1

½ sachet Puffed Sweet & salty Snacks

½ sachet Sharp Cheddar & Sour Cream popcorn

1 teaspoon Parmesan cheese, grated

1 teaspoon sugar-free caramel syrup

1. In a Ziploc bag, place all ingredients.
2. Seal the bag and shake to coat well.
3. Serve immediately.

Cinnamon French Toast Sticks

Prep time: 5 minutes | Cook time: 8 minutes | Serves 2

2 sachets Essential Cinnamon Crunchy O's Cereal

2tablespoons low-fat cream cheese, softened

6 tablespoons liquid egg substitute

Cooking spray

1. Put the Cinnamon Crunchy O's in a blender. Pulse until it has a breadcrumb-like consistency.
2. Pour in the cream cheese and liquid egg substitute, and pulse until a sanity dough forms.
3. Divide and shape the dough into 6 French toast stick pieces.
4. Spritz a skillet with cooking spray. Heat over medium high heat and cook the French toast sticks for 8 minutes on all sides or until lightly browned.
5. Serve immediately.

Chocolate Berry Parfait

Prep time: 10 minutes | Cook time: 0 minutes | Serves 2

1 sachet Chocolate Cherry Ganache Bar

1½ cups low-fat plain Greek yogurt

¼ cup strawberry-flavored light cream cheese, softened

1 tablespoon unsweetened cocoa powder

1 to 2 packets zero-calorie sugar substitute

⅔ ounce (17 g) almonds, sliced

1. In a blender, add all ingredients and pulse until desired consistency is achieved.
2. Serve immediately.

Hearty Zombie Frappe

Prep time: 15 minutes | Cook time: 0 minutes | Serves 1

1 sachet Essential Creamy Vanilla Shake

1 cup unsweetened almond milk

1 tablespoon caramel syrup

½ cup ice

McCormick Color From Nature Food Colors- blue, yellow, and red

2 tablespoons plain, low-fat Greek yogurt

1 tablespoon unsweetened vanilla milk

2 tablespoons pressurized whipped topping

1. Put the Creamy Vanilla Shake, almond milk, caramel syrup, and ice in a blender. Pulse until smooth.
2. Add equal portions of blue and yellow food coloring until the shade of green is achieved.
3. In a bowl, mix the Greek yogurt and equal portions of blue and red food coloring until the shade of purple is achieved.
4. In a separate bowl, mix the vanilla milk with equal portions of blue and red food coloring until the shade of purple is achieved.
5. Drizzle purple Greek yogurt mixture down the sides of a cup. Fill cup with green shake mixture. Top with whipped topping and sprinkle with purple milk mixture.
6. Serve immediately.

Sweet Potato Muffins with Pecans

Prep time: 15 minutes | Cook time: 20 minutes | Serves 4

2 sachets Honey Sweet Potatoes

2 sachets Essential Spiced Gingerbread

¼ cup unsweetened almond milk

6 tablespoons liquid egg substitute

½ teaspoon pumpkin pie spice

½ teaspoon baking powder

½ teaspoon vanilla extract

1 cup water

1½ ounces (43 g) chopped pecans

Cooking Spray

1. Preheat the oven to 350°F (180°C).
2. Cook the Honey Sweet Potatoes according to the package directions. Allow to cool before using.
3. Combine the cooked Honey Sweet Potatoes with remaining ingredients, except for the pecans in a large bowl.
4. Divide the mixture among 8 slots of a greased muffin pan. Sprinkle with pecans on top.
5. Bake in the preheated oven for 20 minutes or until a toothpick inserted in the center comes out clean.
6. Serve immediately.

Tropical Macadamia Smoothie Bowl

Prep time: 10 minutes | Cook time: 0 minutes | Serves 1

1 sachet Essential Tropical Fruit Smoothie

½ cup unsweetened coconut milk

½ cup ice

1 tablespoon shredded, unsweetened coconut

½ ounce (14 g) macadamias, chopped

½ teaspoon lime zest

½ tablespoon chia seeds

1. Add the Tropical Fruit Smoothie, coconut milk, and ice to a blender. Pulse until smooth.
2. Pour the smoothie into a bowl. Spread the remaining ingredients on top and serve.

Maple Pancakes

Prep time: 10 minutes | Cook time: 6 minutes | Serves 1

1 Maple Brown Sugar Oatmeal

¼ teaspoon baking powder

1 tablespoon egg beaters

1 packet stevia

¼ teaspoon ground cinnamon

¼ cup water

1 tablespoon sugar-free pancake syrup

1. In a bowl, add all the ingredients except for pancake syrup and mix until well blended.
2. Heat a lightly greased cast-iron wok over medium-high heat.
3. Place the mixture and with the back of a spoon, spread into a circle.
4. Cook for about 2 to 3 minutes per side or until golden brown.
5. Serve warm with the topping of pancake syrup.

Mac and Cheese Chips

Prep time: 10 minutes | Cook time: 10 minutes | Serves 1

2 packets French Vanilla Shake

1 teaspoon baking powder

1 teaspoon vanilla extract

1 packet Splenda with Fiber

¼ teaspoon ground cinnamon

¼ cup water

1. Preheat the oven to 350°F (180°C).
2. In a blender, add the Mac & Cheese packet and pulse until finely powdered.
3. Transfer the powder into a bowl with water and mix until well blended.
4. Set aside for about 5 minutes.
5. Arrange the dough ball between 2 greased parchment papers and with your hands, flatten into a thin circle.
6. Gently remove the top parchment paper from the dough.
7. Carefully place the dough alongside the parchment paper onto a baking sheet.
8. Bake for approximately 10 minutes.
9. Remove the baking sheet from the oven and with a sharp knife, cut into chips.
10. Arrange the chips onto the baking sheet in a single layer and Bake for approximately 10 minutes or until crispy.
11. Remove the baking sheet of chips from the oven and set aside to cool before serving.

Eggnog

Prep time: 10 minutes | Cook time: 0 minutes | Serves 1

1 sachet Essential Vanilla Shake

8 ounces (227 g) unsweetened almond milk

1 egg (yolk and white separated)

¼ teaspoon rum extract

Pinch of ground nutmeg

1. In a blender, add the Vanilla Shake sachet, almond milk and egg yolk and pulse until smooth.
2. In the bowl of a stand mixer, place egg white and beat on medium speed until stiff peaks form.
3. Place the whipped egg whites into a serving glass and top with Shake mixture.
4. Stir the mixture and sprinkle with nutmeg.
5. Serve immediately.

Mocha Muffin

Prep time: 10 minutes | Cook time: 15 minutes | Serves 4

Muffins:

1 packet Chocolate Chip Pancakes

1 packet Cappuccino

1 tablespoon egg beaters

1 packet stevia powder

¼ teaspoon baking powder

¼ cup water

Frosting:

2 tablespoons light cream cheese, softened

½ packet stevia powder

1. Preheat the oven to 350°F (180°C). Lightly grease 8 cups of a mini muffin tin.
2. For muffins: In a small bowl, add all the ingredients and mix until well combined.
3. Place the mixture into the prepared muffin cups evenly.
4. Bake for approximately 15 minutes or until a toothpick inserted in the center comes out clean.
5. Remove from the oven and place the muffin tin onto a wire rack to cool for about 10 minutes.
6. Carefully invert the muffins onto the wire rack to cool completely before frosting.
7. For frosting: In a small bowl, add the cream cheese and stevia and beat until smooth.
8. Place a dollop of frosting over each muffin and serve.

Pumpkin Frappe

Prep time: 5 minutes | Cook time: 0 minutes | Serves 1

1 sachet Essential Spiced Gingerbread

4 ounces (113 g) strong brewed coffee

4 ounces (113 g) unsweetened almond milk

⅛ teaspoon pumpkin pie spice

½ cup ice

1 tablespoon whipped topping

1. In a blender, add the Spiced Gingerbread sachet, coffee, almond milk, pumpkin pie spice and ice and pulse until smooth.
2. Transfer the mixture into a glass and top with whipped topping.
3. Serve immediately.

Creamy Yogurt Berry Bagels

Prep time: 10 minutes | Cook time: 15 minutes | Serves 2

2 sachets Essential Yogurt Berry Blast Smoothie

2 tablespoons liquid egg substitute

⅓ cup unsweetened almond milk

½ teaspoon baking powder

Cooking spray

1 ounce (28 g) light cream cheese

1. Preheat the oven to 350°F (180°C).
2. In a bowl, mix the Yogurt Berry Blast Smoothie with egg substitute, almond milk, and baking powder.
3. Divide mixture among 4 greased slots of a donut pan.
4. Bake in the preheated oven for 15 minutes or until set.
5. Spread the cream cheese on top and allow to cool before serving.

Rum and Ale Coconut Colada

Prep time: 10 minutes | Cook time: 0 minutes | Serves 1

1 sachet Essential Creamy Vanilla Shake

6 ounces (170 g) unsweetened, original coconut milk

¼ teaspoon rum extract

6 ounces (170 g) diet ginger ale

½ cup ice

2 tablespoons shredded, unsweetened coconut, plus 2 teaspoons for topping

1. Combine all the ingredients in a blender. Pulse until creamy.
2. Divide the mixture among two pina colada glasses. Spread remaining 2 teaspoons of shredded coconut on top.
3. Serve immediately.

Golden Nuggets with Yogurt Dip

Prep time: 10 minutes | Cook time: 18 minutes | Serves 2

12 ounces (340 g) boneless, skinless chicken breast, cubed

2 sachets Essential Honey Mustard and Onion Sticks, crushed into breadcrumb-like consistency

1 egg

¼ cup plain, low-fat Greek yogurt

2 teaspoons spicy brown mustard

¼ teaspoon garlic powder

Cooking Spray

1. Preheat the oven to 400°F (205°C).
2. Pour the crushed Honey Mustard and Onion Sticks in a shallow dish, whisk the egg in another bowl.
3. Dredge the chicken cubes into the egg, and then roll over the crushed Honey Mustard and Onion Sticks until coated. Shake the excess off.
4. Place the chicken cubes on a greased, foil-lined baking sheet. Spritz with cooking spray.
5. Bake in the preheated oven for 18 minutes or until the internal temperature reaches at least 165°F (74°C), flipping halfway through.
6. Meanwhile, to make the yogurt dip, combine the Greek yogurt, mustard, and garlic powder in a small bowl.
7. Serve the chicken nuggets with yogurt dip.

Avocado Toast

Prep time: 5 minutes | Cook time: 15 minutes | Serves 1

1 sachet Buttermilk Cheddar Herb Biscuit

1½ ounces (43 g) avocado, mashed

1. Bake the Buttermilk Cheddar Herb Biscuit according to the package directions.
2. Allow to cool before serving with mashed avocado on top.

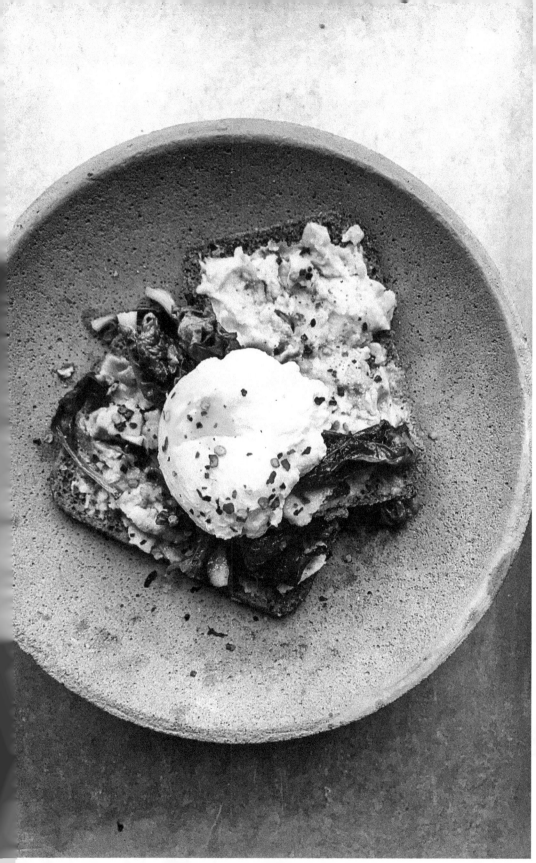

Blueberry Almond Flaxseed Scones

Prep time: 15 minutes | Cook time: 15 minutes | Serves 4

4 sachets Blueberry Almond Hot Cereal

¼ cup ground flaxseeds

2 packets stevia

½ teaspoon baking powder

3 tablespoons unsalted butter, frozen and cut into ½-inch pieces

3 tablespoons liquid egg white

3 tablespoons plain, low-fat Greek yogurt

¼ teaspoon cinnamon

1. Preheat the oven to 400°F (205°C).
2. Add the Blueberry Almond Hot Cereal, ground flaxseeds, stevia, and baking powder to a food processor. Pulse until smooth.
3. Add the frozen butter and pulse until mixture resembles a coarse meal.
4. Add the egg white and Greek yogurt, and pulse until the dough is sanity.
5. Form the dough into a 6-inch circle, then transfer the dough onto a parchment-lined baking sheet. Sprinkle with cinnamon.
6. Bake in the preheated oven for 15 minutes or until lightly browned.
7. After baking, allow to cool before cutting into eight wedges, then serve.

Chia Coconut Pudding

Prep time: 5 minutes | Cook time: 0 minutes | Serves 2

2 sachets Chia Bliss Smoothie

1 cup unsweetened coconut milk

¼ cup chia seeds

1. Combine all the ingredients in a bowl. Stir to mix well.
2. Pour the mixture into a jar and refrigerate overnight.
3. Serve chilled.

Peppermint Mocha

Prep time: 5 minutes | Cook time: 0 minutes | Serves 1

1 sachet Essential Velvety Hot Chocolate

6 ounces (170 g) freshly brewed coffee

¼ cup warm unsweetened almond milk

¼ teaspoon peppermint extract

1 tablespoon whipped topping

Pinch of ground cinnamon

1. In a serving mug, place the Hot Chocolate sachet, coffee, almond milk and peppermint extract and stir until well blended.
2. Top the hot chocolate with whipped topping and sprinkle with cinnamon.
3. Serve immediately.

Crunch Sandwich Cookies

Prep time: 10 minutes | Cook time: 1 minute | Serves 1

1 packet S'more Crunch Bar

1 tablespoon whipped topping

1. Line 2 cups of a muffin tin with cupcake liners.
2. Break the Crunch Bar in 2 pieces.
3. In a microwave-safe bowl, place the bar pieces and microwave for about 15 seconds.
4. Place the bar into the prepared muffin cups evenly and with your fingers press down to form round cookies.
5. Freeze for about 15 minutes.
6. Remove from freezer and place the cookies onto a plate.
7. Spread whipped topping between both cookies and serve.

Cherry Mocha Popsicles

Prep time: 10 minutes | Cook time: 1 minute | Serves 6

1 cup unsweetened almond milk

3 sachets Dark Chocolate Covered Cherry Shake

1 teaspoon vanilla extract

1 tablespoon instant espresso powder

2 cups plain low-fat Greek yogurt

1 to 2 packets zero-calorie sugar substitute

1. In a microwave-safe mug, place the almond milk and microwave on High for about 45 seconds.
2. Remove the mug from microwave and immediately stir in the espresso powder until dissolved completely.
3. Set aside to cool completely.
4. In a blender, add the cooled espresso milk and remaining ingredients and pulse until smooth.
5. Divide the mixture into 6 large Popsicle molds and freeze overnight.

Chocolate Crunch Cookies

Prep time: 10 minutes | Cook time: 2 minutes | Serves 2

1 sachet Brownie Mix

1 Peanut Butter Chocolate Crunch Bar

3 tablespoons water

1. In a bowl, add the brownie mix and water and mix well. Set aside.
2. In a microwave-safe bowl, place the crunch bar and microwave on High for about 20 seconds or until it is slightly melted.
3. Add the crunch bar into the brownie mixture and mix until well combined.
4. Divide the mixture into 2 greased ramekins and microwave on High for about 2 minutes.
5. Remove from microwave and set aside to cool for about 5 minutes before serving.

Chocolate Pumpkin Cheesecake

Prep time: 15 minutes | Cook time: 50 minutes | Serves 1

2 sachets Essential Decadent Double Chocolate Brownie

½ tablespoon unsalted butter, melted

2 tablespoons water

Cooking spray

3 tablespoons pumpkin purée

1 cup nonfat plain Greek yogurt

3 tablespoons light cream cheese, softened

1 egg

½ teaspoon pumpkin pie spice

½ teaspoon vanilla extract

2 packets stevia

Pinch salt

1. Preheat the oven to 350°F (180°C).
2. Combine the Decadent Double Chocolate Brownies, butter, and water in a small bowl.
3. Divide brownie mixture among 2 greased mini springform pans. Press brownie mixture into the bottom. Bake in the preheated oven for 15 minutes.
4. Meanwhile, whisk together the remaining ingredients in a bowl. Divide the mixture among two springform pans.
5. Lower the oven temperature to 300°F (150°C). Bake the cheesecakes for 35 minutes or until lightly browned.
6. Allow to cool before serving.

Vanilla Shake

Prep time: 5 minutes | Cook time: 0 minutes | Serves 1

½ packet Vanilla Shake Fueling

½ packet Gingerbread Fueling

½ cup unsweetened almond milk

½ cup water

8 ice cubes

1. In a small blender, place all ingredients and pulse until smooth.
2. Transfer the shake into a serving glass and serve immediately.

Peanut Butter Cookies

Prep time: 10 minutes | Cook time: 15 minutes | Serves 4

4 sachets Essential Silky Peanut Butter Shake

¼ cup unsweetened almond milk

1 tablespoon butter, melted

¼ teaspoon vanilla extract

¼ teaspoon baking powder

⅛ teaspoon sea salt

Cooking Spray

1. Preheat the oven to 350°F (180°C).
2. Combine all the ingredients, except the sea salt, in a large bowl and keep whisking until a sanity dough forms.

3. Scoop out dough into 8 balls with a cookie scoop. Arrange the balls on a foil-lined, greased baking sheet.

4. Flatten the mounds to create a criss-cross pattern with a fork. Sprinkle with salt.

5. Bake in the preheated oven for 15 minutes or until lightly browned.

6. Serve immediately.

Berry Mojito

Prep time: 10 minutes | Cook time: 0 minutes | Serves 2

2 tablespoons fresh lime juice

6 fresh mint leaves

1 packet Mixed Berry Flavor Infuser

16 ounces (454 g) seltzer water

Ice cubes, as required

1. In the bottom of 2 cocktail glasses, divide the lime juice and mint leaves.

2. With the bottom end of a spoon, gently muddle the mint leaves.

3. Now, divide the Berry Infuser and seltzer water into each glass and stir to combine.

4. Place ice cubes in each glass and serve.

Chocolate Brownie Whoopie

Prep time: 10 minutes | Cook time: 18 minutes | Serves 2

2 sachets Decadent Double Chocolate Brownie

6 tablespoons unsweetened almond milk, divided

3 tablespoons liquid egg substitute

¼ teaspoon baking powder

1 teaspoon vegetable oil

¼ cup powdered peanut butter

Cooking spray

1. Preheat the oven to 350°F (180°C).
2. In a bowl, combine the Decadent Double Chocolate Brownie, ¼ cup almond milk, egg substitute, baking powder, and vegetable oil. Stir to mix well.
3. Divide the Chocolate Brownie batter among 4 slots of a greased muffin tin.
4. Bake in the preheated oven for 18 minutes or until a toothpick inserted in the center comes out clean.
5. Meanwhile, combine the powdered peanut butter and remaining almond milk in a small bowl.
6. When baking is complete, allow to cool, then slice each muffin in half horizontally.
7. Spread 1 tablespoon of peanut butter mixture on the bottom half of each muffin, then top with the remaining muffin halves.
8. Serve immediately.

Turkey Bacon Savory Potato Waffles

Prep time: 10 minutes | Cook time: 6 minutes | Serves 4

4 sachets Essential Roasted Garlic Creamy Smashed Potatoes

½ cup unsweetened almond milk

½ cup shredded, reduced-fat Cheddar cheese

½ cup liquid egg substitute

2 slices turkey bacon, cooked and chopped into small pieces

¼ cup chopped scallions

Cooking spray

1. Mix the Garlic Creamy Smashed Potatoes, almond milk, Cheddar cheese, and egg substitute in a bowl, then stir in the remaining ingredients.
2. Pour the mixture on a greased waffle iron. Close the lid and bake for 6 minutes or until lightly browned.
3. Serve immediately.

Caramel Macchiato Frappe

Prep time: 10 minutes | Cook time: 0 minutes | Serves 1

8 ounces (227 g) unsweetened cashew milk

1 sachet Essential Caramel Macchiato Shake

½ cup ice

2 tablespoons whipped topping

1 tablespoon sugar-free caramel syrup

1. In a blender, add the Macchiato Shake sachet, cashew milk and ice and pulse until smooth.

2. Transfer the mixture into a glass and top with whipped topping.

3. Drizzle with caramel syrup and serve immediately.

Mini Biscuit Pizza

Prep time: 10 minutes | Cook time: 14 minutes | Serves 1

1 sachet Buttermilk Cheddar and Herb Biscuit

2 tablespoons water

1 tablespoon tomato sauce

1 tablespoon low-fat Cheddar cheese, shredded

1. Preheat the oven to 350°F (180°C).

2. In a small bowl, add the biscuit and water and mix well.

3. Place the biscuit mixture onto a parchment paper and with a spoon, spread into a thin circle.

4. Bake for approximately 10 minutes.

5. Remove from the oven and spread the tomato sauce over the biscuit circle.

6. Sprinkle with Cheddar cheese.

7. Bake for approximately 2 to 4 minutes or until cheese is melted.

8. Remove from the oven and set aside for about 3 to 5 minutes.

9. Serve warm.

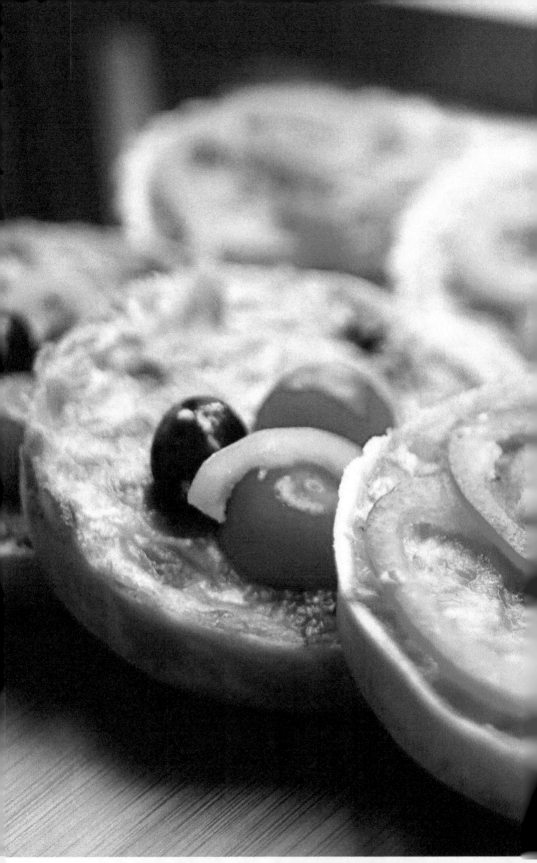

10.

Chocolate Shake

Prep time: 10 minutes | Cook time: 0 minutes | Serves 1

1 packet cappuccino mix

½ cup water

1 tablespoon sugar-free chocolate syrup

½ cup ice, crushed

1. In a small blender, place all ingredients and pulse until smooth.
2. Transfer the shake into a serving glass and serve immediately.

Caramel Crunch Parfait

Prep time: 10 minutes | Cook time: 0 minutes | Serves 1

6 ounces (170 g) low-fat plain Greek yogurt

½ packet stevia

¼ teaspoon vanilla extract

2 tablespoons whipped topping

1 sachet Puffed Sweet & Salty Snacks, crushed

1 tablespoon sugar-free caramel syrup

1. In a bowl, mix together the yogurt, stevia and vanilla extract.
2. Top with whipped topping Puffed Snack sachet.
3. Drizzle with caramel syrup and serve.

Snickerdoodles

Prep time: 10 minutes | Cook time: 8 minutes | Serves 2

2 packets French Vanilla Shake

1 packet Splenda with Fiber

1 teaspoon baking powder

¼ teaspoon ground cinnamon

1 teaspoon vanilla extract

¼ cup water

1. Preheat the oven to 350°F (180°C). Line a cookie sheet with parchment paper.
2. In a bowl, add the Vanilla Shake packet, Splenda, baking powder and cinnamon and mix well.
3. Add the vanilla extract and mix well.
4. Slowly, add the water and mix until a paste is formed.
5. With a spoon, place 4 cookies onto the prepared cookie sheet in a single layer and with your fingers, press each ball slightly.
6. Bake for approximately 8 minutes.
7. Remove from oven and place the cookie sheet onto a wire rack to cool for about 5 minutes.
8. Now, invert the cookies onto the wire rack to cool before serving.

Marshmallow Cereal Treat

Prep time: 5 minutes | Cook time: 1 minute | Serves 1

1 packet Meal Mixed Berry Cereal Crunch

2 tablespoons marshmallow dip

1. In a small bowl, add the Cereal Crunch and marshmallow dip and mix well.
2. Place the mixture into a microwave-safe mini loaf pan and with the back of a spoon, press slightly.
3. Microwave for about 1 minute.
4. Remove from the microwave and set aside to cool completely before serving.

Chocolate Crepe

Prep time: 10 minutes | Cook time: 4 minutes | Serves 1

1 packet Chocolate Chip Pancakes

¼ cup water

¼ cup part-skim ricotta cheese

½ packet stevia powder

⅛ teaspoon vanilla extract

1 teaspoon sugar-free chocolate syrup

1. In a bowl, add the pancake and water and mix well.
2. Heat a lightly greased skillet over medium heat.
3. Place the mixture and spread in a thin circle.
4. Cook for about 1 to 2 minutes per side or until golden brown.
5. Remove from the heat and place the crepe onto a plate.

6. In a small bowl, add the ricotta cheese, stevia and vanilla extract and mix until well combined.

7. Place the mixture inside the crepe.

8. Drizzle with chocolate syrup and serve.

Quick Mint Cookies

Prep time: 10 minutes | Cook time: 15 minutes | Serves 4

2 sachets Essential Decadent Double Chocolate Brownie

2 sachets Essential Chocolate Mint Cookie Crisp Bars, softened

2 tablespoons unsweetened almond milk

1 tablespoon liquid egg substitute

¼ teaspoon mint extract

1. Preheat the oven to 350°F (180°C).

2. In a small bowl, whisk together the Decadent Double Chocolate Brownies, almond milk, egg substitute, and mint extract. Stir in the microwave crunch bars until the bars break into tiny pieces.

3. Form the mixture into eight cookie, then arrange the cookies on a parchment-lined baking sheet

4. Bake in the preheated oven for 15 minutes or until set and lightly browned.

5. Serve immediately.

Brownie Bites

Prep time: 10 minutes | Cook time: 0 minutes | Serves 6

3 tablespoons peanut butter powder

1 cup plus 3 tablespoons water, divided

6 sachets Double Chocolate Brownie Mix

1 cup water

1. In a small bowl, add the peanut butter powder and 3 tablespoons of water and mix until well combined.
2. In another bowl, add Double Chocolate Brownie sachets and remaining water and mix until well combined.
3. In the bottom of 6 silicon molds, place the peanut butter powder mixture evenly and top with brownie mixture.
4. Freeze the molds until set completely.
5. Remove from the freezer and set aside for about 30 to 40 minutes before serving.

Pumpkin Gingerbread Latte

Prep time: 5 minutes | Cook time: 1 minutes | Serves 1

2 tablespoons pumpkin purée

½ cup unsweetened almond milk

1 sachet Essential Spiced Gingerbread

½ cup strong brewed coffee

1. Combine the pumpkin purée and milk in a microwave-safe mug. Microwave for 1 minute and stir.
2. Mix in the coffee and Spiced Gingerbread. Serve immediately.

Meringue Cups

Prep time: 10 minutes | Cook time: 3 minutes | Serves 2

2 Essential Zesty lemon Crisp Bars, crushed roughly

1 ½ cups low-fat plain Greek yogurt

1 (0.3-ounce / 9-g) box sugar-free lemon gelatin

½ teaspoon lime zest, grated

1. Line 6 cups of a muffin tin with paper liners.
2. In a microwave-safe bowl, place Crisp Bar sachets and microwave for about 10 to 15 seconds.
3. Divide the crisp bar pieces into the prepared muffin cups evenly.
4. In another microwave-safe bowl, place yogurt and gelatin and microwave for about 2 minutes, stirring after every 40 seconds.
5. Remove from microwave and stir until smooth.
6. Place the yogurt mixture over crunch bar I each muffin cup.
7. Refrigerate for at least 1 hour before serving.
8. Garnish with lime zest and serving.

Brownie Peanut Butter Pudding

Prep time: 5 minutes | Cook time: 0 minutes | Serves 1

1 packet Brownie

1 (5.3-ounce / 150-g) container low-fat plain Greek yogurt

1 tablespoon peanut butter powder

Dash of vanilla extract

1. In a bowl, add all ingredients and mix until well combined.
2. Refrigerate to chill before serving.

Mini Chocolate Cakes

Prep time: 10 minutes | Cook time: 18 minutes | Serves 2

1 packet Chocolate Chip Pancakes

1 sachet Brownie Mix

¼ teaspoon baking powder

¼ cup water

1. Preheat the oven to 350°F (180°C). Grease 2 cups of a muffin tin.
2. In a bowl, add all the ingredients and mix until well combined.
3. Place the mixture into the prepared muffin cups evenly.
4. Bake for approximately 18 minutes or until a toothpick inserted in the center comes out clean.
5. Remove from the oven and place the muffin tin onto a wire rack to cool for about 10 minutes.

6. Carefully invert the muffins onto the wire rack to cool completely before serving.

Peanut Butter Bites

Prep time: 10 minutes | Cook time: 1 minute | Serves 1

2 tablespoons peanut butter powder

1 tablespoon water

1 sachet Essential Creamy Double Peanut Butter Crisp Bar

1. In a bowl, add the peanut butter powder and water and mix until a smooth paste is formed.
2. In a microwave-safe plate, place the Crisp Bar and microwave for about 15 seconds or until soft.
3. Add the warm bar pieces into the bowl of water mixture and mix until a dough forms.
4. Make small 4 equal-sized balls from the dough and arrange onto a parchment paper-lined plate.
5. Refrigerate until set before serving.

Cinnamon Buns

Prep time: 5 minutes | Cook time: 1 minute | Serves 1

1 Pancake Mix

1 packet Splenda

¼ teaspoon ground cinnamon

⅛ teaspoon baking powder

2 tablespoons water

¼ teaspoon vanilla extract

1. In a bowl, add all ingredients and mix until well combined.
2. Place the mixture into a greased microwave-safe bowl and sprinkle with extra cinnamon.
3. Microwave for about 50 to 60 seconds.
4. Serve warm.

Parmesan Chicken Bites

Prep time: 15 minutes | Cook time: 30 minutes | Serves 3

2 packets Parmesan Cheese Puffs, crushed finely

2 ounces (57 g) boneless, skinless chicken breast, cubed

2 tablespoons low-fat Parmesan cheese, grated

2 tablespoons hot sauce

1. Preheat the oven to 350°F (180°C).
2. Line a baking sheet with parchment paper.
3. In a plastic Ziploc bag, place the crushed Parmesan puffs and Parmesan cheese and mix well.
4. In a bowl, add chicken cubes and hot sauce and toss to coat well.
5. Place the coated chicken cubes in the bag with Parmesan mixture.
6. Seal the bag and shake to coat well.
7. Arrange the coated chicken cubes onto the prepared baking sheet in a single layer.
8. Bake for approximately 25 to 30 minutes.
9. Serve warm.

Mac and Cheese Waffles

Prep time: 10 minutes | Cook time: 10 minutes | Serves 2

2 packets Chipotle Mac & Cheese

6 tablespoons liquid egg whites

4 ounces (113 g) cold water

2 tablespoons sugar-free maple syrup

1. In a microwave-safe bowl, place Mac & Cheese packets and water and mix well.
2. Microwave on high for about 1 to 1½ minutes. Remove from microwave and stir well.
3. Set aside for about 1 minute.
4. Microwave on high for about 1 minute.
5. Remove from microwave and stir well. Set aside until cooled.
6. Add liquid egg whites and stir to combine.
7. Preheat a waffle iron and then grease it.
8. Place the mixture into the preheated waffle iron and cook for about 5 to 7 minutes or until golden brown.
9. Repeat with the remaining mixture.
10. Serve warm with the topping of maple syrup.

Fudge Balls

Prep time: 10 minutes | Cook time: 0 minutes | Serves 2

1 sachet chocolate pudding

1 sachet chocolate shake

4 tablespoons peanut butter powder

¼ cup unsweetened almond milk

2 tablespoons water

1. In a small bowl, add all the ingredients and mix until well combined.
2. Make 8 small equal-sized balls from the mixture.
3. Arrange the balls onto a parchment paper-lined baking sheet and refrigerate until set before serving.

Shamrock Shake

Prep time: 5 minutes | Cook time: 0 minutes | Serves 1

1 packet Vanilla Shake

6 ounces (170 g) unsweetened almond milk

¼ teaspoon peppermint extract

1 to 2 drops green food coloring

1 cup ice cubes

1. In a small blender, place all ingredients and pulse until smooth.
2. Transfer the shake into a serving glass and serve immediately.

Pizza Bread

Prep time: 10 minutes | Cook time: 10 minutes | Serves 1

1 packet Cream of Tomato Soup

¼ teaspoon baking powder

Salt and ground black pepper, to taste

2 tablespoons water

¼ cup low-fat Cheddar cheese, shredded

1. Preheat the oven to 425°F (220°C). Grease a small baking sheet.
2. In a bowl, add the soup, baking powder, salt, black pepper and water and mix until well combined.
3. Place the mixture onto the prepared baking sheet and shape into a circle.
4. Bake for approximately 5 minutes.
5. Remove from the oven and with a spatula, flip the bread.
6. Top with the cheese and Bake for approximately 5 minutes more.
7. Serve warm.

Blueberry Muffins

Prep time: 10 minutes | Cook time: 10 minutes | Serves 6

6 packets Wild Blueberry Almond Hot Cereal

1½ tablespoons baking powder

¾ cup water

¾ cup liquid egg substitute

1. Preheat the oven to 350ºF (180ºC).
2. Grease 6 holes of a mini muffin tin.
3. In a bowl, place all ingredients and mix well.
4. Place the mixture into the prepared muffin cups evenly.
5. Bake for approximately 10 minutes or until a toothpick inserted in the center comes out clean.
6. Remove the muffin tin from oven and place onto a wire rack to cool for about 10 minutes.
7. Carefully invert the muffins onto the wire rack to cool completely before serving.

Mac and Cheese Doritos

Prep time: 15 minutes | Cook time: 15 minutes | Serves 1

1 packet Macaroni & Cheese

¼ teaspoon garlic salt

¼ teaspoon red pepper flakes, crushed

2 tablespoons water

Pinch of red chili powder

cooking spray

1. Preheat the oven to 350ºF (180ºC).
2. In a food processor, add mac & cheese packet, garlic salt and red pepper flakes and pulse until finely powdered.
3. Transfer into a bowl with water and stir to combine.
4. Set aside for about 2 minutes.

5. Place the dough between 2 greased pieces of parchment and with your hands, spread into a thin circle.

6. Carefully peel off the top layer of parchment.

7. Arrange the dough onto a baking sheet alongside the parchment paper.

8. Sprinkle the dough with chili powder.

9. Bake for approximately 10 minutes.

10. Remove from the oven and with a pizza cutter, cut into chip-size pieces.

11. Flip the chips and Bake for approximately 3 to 5 minutes.

12. Remove from the oven and set aside to cool completely before serving.

Marshmallow Cereal Cake

Prep time: 5 minutes | Cook time: 1 minute | Serves 1

1 packet Meal Mixed Berry Cereal Crunch

2 tablespoons marshmallow dip

1. In a small bowl, add the Cereal Crunch and marshmallow dip and mix well.

2. Place the mixture into a microwave-safe mini loaf pan and with the back of a spoon, press slightly.

3. Microwave for about 1 minute.

4. Remove from the microwave and set aside to cool completely before serving.

Noodle Soup Chips

Prep time: 15 minutes | Cook time: 18 minutes | Serves 1

1 packet Chicken Noodle Soup

3 tablespoons water

Olive oil cooking spray

1. Preheat the oven to 375°F (190°C).
2. In a small blender, add the soup sachet and pulse powdered finely.
3. In a small bowl, add the powdered soup and water and mix until dough ball forms.
4. Set aside for about 3 to 5 minutes.
5. Arrange the dough ball between 2 grease parchment papers and with your hands, flatten into a thinner circle.
6. Carefully remove the parchment paper from the top of the dough.
7. Carefully place the parchment paper with dough onto a baking sheet.
8. Bake for approximately 10 minutes.
9. Remove the baking sheet from the oven and with a sharp knife, cut into chips.
10. Arrange the chips onto the baking sheet in a single layer and Bake for approximately 6 to 8 minutes or until crispy.
11. Remove from the oven and set aside to cool before serving.

Taco Salad

Prep time: 10 minutes | Cook time: 0 minutes | Serves 1

5 ounces (142 g) cooked extra-lean ground turkey

2 cups romaine lettuce, shredded

½ medium orange bell pepper, seeded and chopped

¼ cup low-fat Mexican blend cheese, shredded

2 tablespoons pico de gallo

2 tablespoons lime vinaigrette

1 sachet Puffed Ranch Snack

1.   In a bowl, place turkey, lettuce, bell pepper, cheese and pico de gallo and mix well.
2.   Drizzle with vinaigrette.
3.   Top with Ranch Snack sachet and serve.

Coconut Smoothie

Prep time: 5 minutes | Cook time: 0 minutes | Serves 1

1 sachet Essential Creamy Vanilla Shake

6 ounces (170 g) unsweetened almond milk

6 ounces (170 g) diet ginger ale

2 tablespoons unsweetened coconut, shredded

¼ teaspoon rum extract

½ cup ice

1.   In a small blender, place all ingredients and pulse until smooth.

2. Transfer the smoothie into a serving glass and serve immediately.

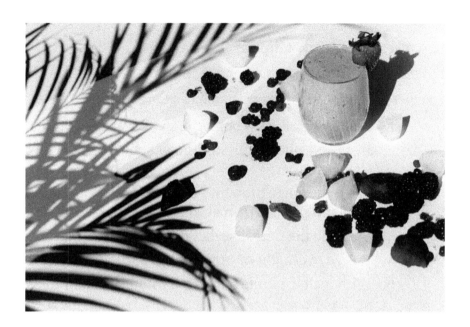

Yogurt Cereal Bark

Prep time: 10 minutes | Cook time: 0 minutes | Serves 2

12 ounces (340 g) low-fat plain Greek yogurt

1 to 2 packets zero-calorie sugar substitute

1 sachet Essential Red Berry Crunch O's Cereal

1. Line an 8 × 8-inch baking dish with a piece of foil.
2. In a bowl, add yogurt and sugar substitute and mix well.
3. Place the yogurt mixture into the prepared baking dish and spread in an even layer.
4. Sprinkle the Cereal sachet on top evenly.
5. Freeze overnight or until bark is hard.
6. With a sharp knife, cut the bark into small pieces and serve.

Pumpkin Waffles

Prep time: 10 minutes | Cook time: 8 minutes | Serves 2

1 sachet Golden Pancake

1 tablespoon 100% canned pumpkin

¼ teaspoon pumpkin pie spice

Pinch of ground cinnamon

¼ cup water

2 tablespoons sugar-free pancake syrup

1. Preheat a mini waffle iron and then grease it.

2. In a bowl, add all ingredients except for pancake syrup and mix until well blended.
3. Place ½ of the mixture into the preheated waffle iron and cook for about 3 to 4 minutes or until golden brown.
4. Repeat with the remaining mixture.
5. Serve warm with the topping of pancake syrup.

Tortilla Chips

Prep time: 10 minutes | Cook time: 25 minutes | Serves 2

2 sachets Hearty Red Bean & Vegetable Chili

¼ cup water

1. Preheat the oven to 350°F (180°C).
2. Line a rimmed baking sheet with a lightly greased parchment paper.
3. In a food processor, add the Vegetable Chili sachet and pulse until finely powdered.
4. Transfer the Vegetable Chili powder into a bowl with water and beat until smooth.
5. Arrange the dough onto the prepared baking sheet and with your hands, smooth the top surface.
6. With a knife, cut the dough into chips pieces.
7. Bake for approximately 10 minutes.
8. Carefully flip the dough pieces and Bake for approximately 10 to 15 minutes.
9. Remove the baking sheet of chips from the oven and set aside to cool before serving.

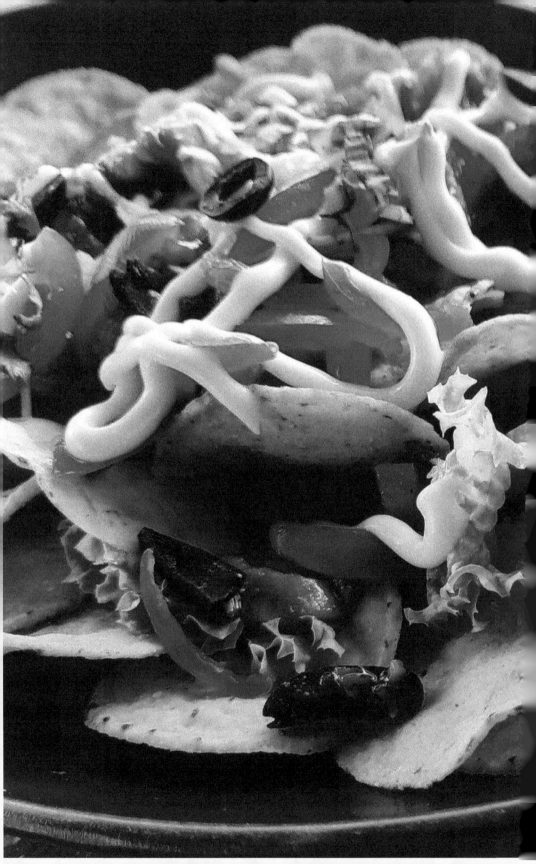

10.

Sriracha Popcorn

Prep time: 5 minutes | Cook time: 0 minutes | Serves 1

1 teaspoon unsalted butter, melted

1 teaspoon Sriracha

Pinch of stevia powder

1 sachet Sharp Cheddar & Sour Cream Popcorn

1. In a Ziploc bag, place all ingredients.
2. Seal the bag and shake to coat well.
3. Serve immediately.

Potato Bagels

Prep time: 10 minutes | Cook time: 12 minutes | Serves 1

2 egg whites

1 sachet Mashed Potatoes

1 teaspoon baking powder

1. Preheat the oven to 350°F (180°C).
2. Lightly grease 1 hole of a donut pan.
3. In a bowl, add the egg whites and beat until foamy.
4. Add the baking powder and mashed potatoes and beat until well blended.
5. Place the mixture into the prepare donut hole.
6. Bake for approximately 10 to 12 minutes or until done.
7. Serve warm.

Cheesy Smashed Potato

Prep time: 5 minutes | Cook time: 12 minutes | Serves 2

2 sachets Essential Smashed Potatoes

1 cup water

1 cup reduced fat, shredded Mozzarella cheese

1. In a microwave-safe bowl, mix the Essential Smashed Potatoes and water to combine well.
2. Microwave on high for 1½ minutes, then stir.
3. Pour the mixture into a lightly greased waffle iron. Close lid and cook for 10 minutes or until lightly browned.
4. Open the lid and sprinkle with the cheese on one half of the waffle. Fold over the other half of the waffle.
5. Close the lid and continue cooking for 2 minutes or until cheese melts.
6. Serve immediately.

Chocolate Waffles

Prep time: 10 minutes | Cook time: 8 minutes | Serves 2

1 packet Chocolate Chip Pancakes

¼ teaspoon pumpkin pie spice

1 tablespoon 100% canned pumpkin

¼ cup water

2 teaspoons sugar-free pancake syrup

1. Preheat a mini waffle iron and then grease it.

2. In a bowl, add all the ingredients except for pancake syrup and mix until well combined.
3. Place ½ of the mixture into preheated waffle iron and cook for about 3 to 4 minutes or until golden brown.
4. Repeat with the remaining mixture.
5. Serve warm with the topping of pancake syrup

Buffalo Cauliflower Poppers

Prep time: 15 minutes | Cook time: 30 minutes | Serves 3

1 sachets Cheddar Herb Biscuit

¼ cup hot buffalo sauce

½ cup water

3 cups cauliflower florets

½ tablespoons butter, melted

1. Preheat the oven to 425°F (220°C).
2. Line a large baking sheet with a lightly greased piece of foil.
3. In a bowl, add the Biscuit sachet and water and mix until well combined.
4. Add the cauliflower florets and toss to coat well.
5. Arrange the cauliflower florets onto the prepared baking sheet in a single layer.
6. Bake for approximately 20 minutes.
7. Meanwhile, in a bowl, add the buffalo sauce and butter and mix well.
8. Remove the baking sheet from oven.
9. In the bowl of sauce mixture, add the cauliflower florets and toss to coat well.

10. Again arrange the cauliflower florets onto the same baking sheet in a single layer.

11. Bake for approximately 7 to 10 minutes. Serve warm.

Chocolate Donuts

Prep time: 15 minutes | Cook time: 27 minutes | Serves 4

2 sachets Essential Decadent Double Brownie

2 sachets Essential Chocolate Chip Pancakes

6 tablespoons liquid egg substitute

¼ cup unsweetened almond milk

½ teaspoon vanilla extract

½ teaspoon baking powder

1. Preheat the oven to 350°F (180°C). Lightly grease 4 holes of a donut pan.

2. In a bowl, add all ingredients and mix until well blended.

3. Place the mixture into the prepared donut pan evenly.

4. Bake for approximately 12 to 15 minutes or until donuts are set completely.

5. Remove from the oven and set aside to cool slightly.

6. Serve warm.

Yogurt Berry Donuts

Prep time: 10 minutes | Cook time: 15 minutes | Serves 2

2 sachets Yogurt Berry Blast Smoothie

2 tablespoons liquid egg substitute

⅓ cup unsweetened almond milk

½ teaspoon baking powder

Olive oil cooking spray

1. Preheat the oven to 350°F (180°C).
2. Lightly grease 4 holes of a donut pan.
3. In a bowl, add the Smoothie sachets, milk, egg substitute and baking powder and mix well.
4. Divide the mixture into the prepared donut holes.
5. Bake for approximately 12 to 15 minutes.
6. Remove from the oven and set aside to cool slightly before serving.

Gingersnap Cookies

Prep time: 10 minutes | Cook time: 20 minutes | Serves 1

1 sachet Essential Spiced Gingerbread

2 tablespoons cold water

Olive oil cooking spray

2 tablespoons low-fat whipped cream cheese spread

⅛ teaspoon vanilla tract

3 to 5 drops liquid stevia

1. Preheat the oven to 350°F (180°C).

2. Lightly grease a cookie sheet.

3. In a bowl, add Spiced Gingerbread sachet and beat until smooth.

4. With a small spoon, place about 3 cookies onto the prepared cookie sheet in a single layer.

5. Bake for approximately 18 to 20 minutes or until golden brown.

6. Remove from the oven and place the cookie sheet onto a wire rack to cool for about 5 minutes.

7. Now, invert the cookies onto the wire rack to cool before serving.

8. Meanwhile, in a small bowl, place cream cheese, vanilla extract and stevia and beat until smooth.

9. Spread frosting over cookies and serve.

Chocolate Cake Fries

Prep time: 10 minutes | Cook time: 4 minutes | Serves 2

2 sachets essential Golden Chocolate Chip Pancakes

¼ cup liquid egg substitute

2 teaspoons vegetable oil

1. In a bowl, add Pancakes sachets and egg substitute and mix until well combined.

2. Place the mixture into a resealable plastic bag.

3. Cut off a small hole on tip of the bag.

4. In a skillet, heat oil over medium heat.

5. In the skillet, pipe mixture in long, straight lines and cook for about 2 minutes per side.

6. Serve warm.

Peanut Butter Cups

Prep time: 15 minutes | Cook time: 0 minutes | Serves 4

2 sachets Essential Decadent Double Chocolate Brownie

9 to 10 tablespoons unsweetened almond milk, divided

¼ cup powdered peanut butter

1. In a small bowl, add the brownie sachet and 6 tablespoons of almond milk and mix well.
2. In another bowl, add the remaining milk and peanut butter powder and mix well.
3. In 2 different pipping bags, place the brownie mixture and peanut butter powder mixture respectively.
4. In the bottom of 20 silicone baking molds, place the brownie mixture about ⅓ way of full.
5. Top each mold with a little peanut butter powder mixture.
6. Place the remaining brownie mixture on top evenly.
7. Freeze for at least 2 hours before serving.

Hot Chocolate

Prep time: 10 minutes | Cook time: 2 minutes | Serves 1

1 sachet Essential Velvety Hot Chocolate

½ teaspoon ground cinnamon

Pinch of cayenne pepper

6 ounces (170 g) unsweetened almond milk

1 tablespoon whipped cream

1. In a serving mug, place all the ingredients except for whipped cream and beat until well blended.
2. Microwave on high for about 2 minutes.
3. Top with whipped cream and serve.

Shake Cake

Prep time: 10 minutes | Cook time: 15 minutes | Serves 1

1 packet Shake

¼ teaspoon baking powder

2 tablespoons water

2 tablespoons egg beaters

1. Preheat the oven to 350°F (180°C). Lightly grease a ramekin.
2. In a bowl, add all the ingredients and mix until well combined.
3. Place the mixture into the prepared ramekin.
4. Bake for approximately 15 minutes.
5. Remove the ramekin from oven and place onto a wire rack to cool for about 10 minutes.
6. Carefully invert the cake onto the wire rack to cool completely before serving.

Oatmeal Cookies

Prep time: 10 minutes | Cook time: 15 minutes | Serves 2

1 oatmeal raisin crunch bar

1 packet oatmeal

⅛ teaspoon ground cinnamon

1 packet stevia powder

⅛ teaspoon baking powder

½ teaspoon vanilla extract

⅓ cup water

1. Preheat the oven to 350°F (180°C). Line a cookie sheet with parchment paper.
2. In a microwave-safe bowl, place the crunch bar and microwave on High for about 15 seconds or until it is slightly melted.
3. In the bowl of bar, add the remaining ingredients and mix until well combined.
4. Set the mixture aside for about 5 minutes.
5. With a spoon, place 4 cookies onto the prepared cookie sheet in a single layer and with your fingers, press each ball slightly.
6. Bake for approximately 12 to 15 minutes or until golden brown.
7. Remove from oven and place the cookie sheet onto a wire rack to cool for about 5 minutes.
8. Now, invert the cookies onto the wire rack to cool before serving.

Chocolate Frappe

Prep time: 5 minutes | Cook time: 0 minutes | Serves 1

1 sachet Essential Frosty Mint Chocolate Soft Serve Treat

4 ounces (113 g) strong brewed coffee

4 ounces (113 g) unsweetened almond milk

1½ tablespoons sugar-free chocolate syrup, divided

¼ teaspoon peppermint extract

½ cup ice

1 tablespoon whipped topping

1. In a blender, add the Chocolate sachet, coffee, almond milk, 1 tablespoon of chocolate syrup, peppermint extract and ice and pulse until smooth.
2. Transfer the mixture into a glass and top with whipped topping.
3. Drizzle with remaining chocolate syrup and serve immediately.

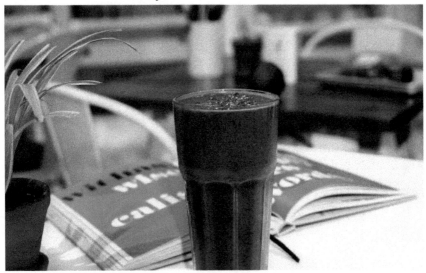

Oatmeal Waffles

Prep time: 5 minutes | Cook time: 12 minutes | Serves 1

1 packet Oatmeal

½ teaspoon baking powder

2 tablespoons egg whites

½ teaspoon vanilla extract

Pinch of Molly McButter

Pinch of ground cinnamon

½ cup cold water

2 tablespoons sugar-free maple syrup

1. Preheat a waffle iron and then grease it.
2. In a bowl, add all ingredients except for maple syrup and mix until well blended.
3. Place the mixture into the preheated waffle iron and cook for 6 to 7 minutes.
4. Carefully flip the waffle and cook for about 5 minutes or until golden brown.
5. Repeat with the remaining mixture.
6. Serve warm with the topping of maple syrup.

Simple Yogurt Chocolate Cookie Dough

Prep time: 5 minutes | Cook time: 0 minutes | Serves 1

1 sachet Essential Chewy Chocolate Chip Cookie

1 (5.3-ounce / 150-g) container low-fat plain Greek yogurt

1. Combine the Chewy Chocolate Chip Cookie with the Greek yogurt in a bowl.
2. Chill until ready to serve.

Cheese and Tomato Caprese Pizza Bites

Prep time: 10 minutes | Cook time: 12 minutes | Serves 4

4 sachets Buttermilk Cheddar Herb Biscuit

½ cup unsweetened almond milk

2 teaspoons olive oil

1 cup basil leaves, julienned

4 ounces (113 g) fresh Mozzarella log, cut into 12 small pieces

3 Roma tomatoes, thinly sliced

2 tablespoons balsamic vinegar

Cooking spray

1. Preheat the oven to 450°F (235°C).
2. In a bowl, mix Buttermilk Cheddar Herb Biscuit, almond milk, and olive oil until well combined.
3. Divide the biscuit mixture among 12 slots of a greased muffin tin.
4. Layer a slice of Mozzarella, then a slice of tomato, and then a few pieces of basil into each slot.
5. Bake in the preheated oven for 12 minutes or until biscuit mixture is well browned and cheese is bubbly.
6. Drizzle with balsamic vinegar on top before serving.

Pumpkin Pie Trail Mix

Prep time: 10 minutes | Cook time: 0 minutes | Serves 1

1 sachet Olive Oil & Sea Salt Popcorn

½ tablespoon pumpkin seeds

½ tablespoon slivered almonds

½ tablespoon sugar-free pancake syrup

¼ teaspoon pumpkin pie spice

1. In a Ziploc bag, place all ingredients.
2. Seal the bag and shake to coat well.
3. Serve immediately.

Tiramisu Shake

Prep time: 5 minutes | Cook time: 0 minutes | Serves 1

1 packet cappuccino mix

1 tablespoon sugar-free chocolate syrup

½ cup water

½ cup ice, crushed

1. In a small blender, add all the ingredients and pulse until smooth and creamy.
2. Transfer the shake into a serving glass and serve immediately.

Mocha Cake

Prep time: 5 minutes | Cook time: 2 minutes | Serves 2

1 packet Calorie Burn Cappuccino

1 packet Chocolate Chip Pancakes

1 packet Splenda

1 tablespoon egg beaters

¼ teaspoon baking powder

¼ cup water

1. In a bowl, add all ingredients and stir until well blended.
2. Place the mixture into a greased 4-inch round microwave-safe dish and microwave on High for about 1¾ to 2 minutes.
3. Remove from the microwave and divide into 2 portions.
4. Serve warm.

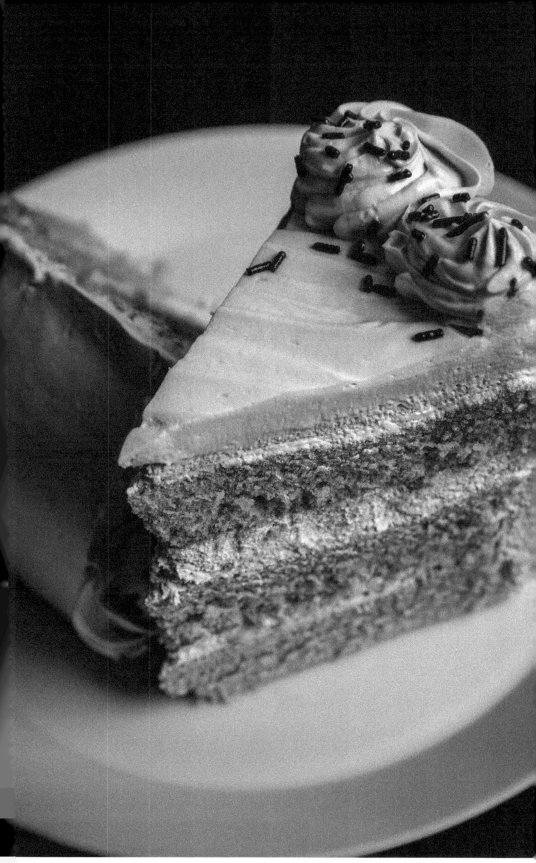

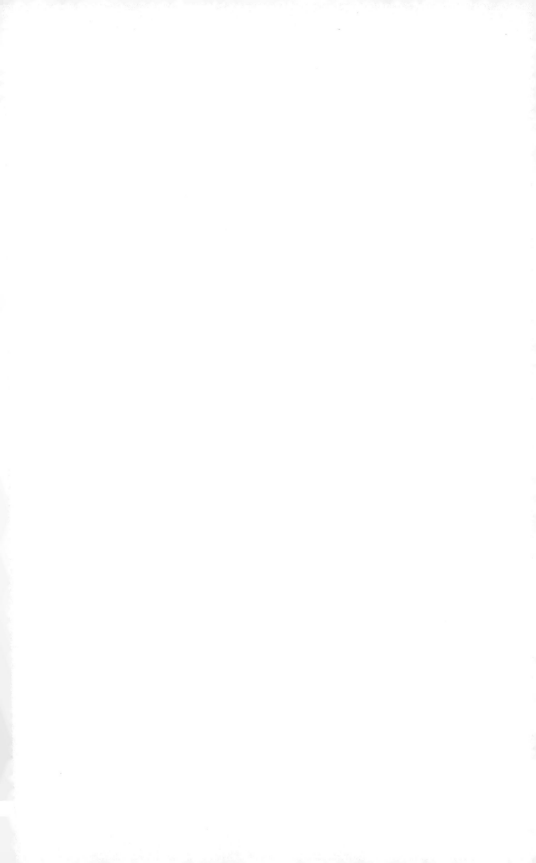

Lightning Source UK Ltd.
Milton Keynes UK
UKHW020657310521
384668UK00001B/104